HOW TO LIVE

WITH

SCHIZOPHRENIA

HOW TO LIVE WITH SCHIZOPHRENIA

New Revised Edition

by

Abram Hoffer, M.D., Ph.D.

and

Humphry Osmond, M.R.C.S., D.P.M.

With a Foreword by Nolen D. C. Lewis, M. D.

A Citadel Press Book
Published by Carol Publishing Group

PUBLISHER'S NOTE

This book is written for schizophrenics and their families and the interested lay public. Hence it usually provides none of the references to page and chapter in the medical literature. Those who wish to know the scientific literature relating to the subject of this book may consult the following work: NIACIN THERAPY AND PSYCHIATRY, by Abram Hoffer, Ph.D., M.D., published by Charles C. Thomas, Springfield, Illinois. This book gives the results of the clinical trial of massive does of niacin on schizophrenics begun in 1952. Over one hundred case histories are cited.

A Citadel Press Book
Published by Carol Publishing Group
Citadel Press is a registered trademark of Carol Communications, Inc.

Editorial Offices: 600 Madison Avenue, New York, N.Y. 10022
Sales & Distribution Offices: 120 Enterprise Avenue, Secaucus, N.J. 07094
In Canada: Canadian Manda Group, P.O. Box 920, Station U, Toronto, Ontario M8Z 5P9

Queries regarding rights and permissions should be addressed to Carol Publishing Group, 600 Madison Avenue, New York, N.Y. 10022

Carol Publishing Group books are available at special discounts for bulk purchases, for sales promotions, fund raising, or educational purposes. Special editions can be created to specifications. For details contact: Special Sales Department, Carol Publishing Group, 120 Enterprise Avenue, Secaucus, N.J. 07094

Manufactured in the United States of America
10 9 8 7 6 5 4 3 2 1

ISBN 0-8065-1382-9

CONTENTS

FOREWORD

THIS is a unique book in two ways. It is the first book written for the schizophrenic and schizoid patients, instructing them in what attitude they should take to live with the disorder. Secondly, the authors have accomplished the difficult task of presenting a longitudinal picture of the whole problem in perspective, utilizing only those terms that can be readily understood by the general reader.

The authors' description of the nature of the disorder, including its universality, inheritance aspects, physical and physiological changes and psychological phenomena, such as changes in thought processes, mood changes, behavior oddities and numerous examples of depersonalization phenomena, afford the necessary orientation desirable to approach the more complicated items and theories concerning causes described in subsequent sections of the text. Biochemical, psychological and sociological factors are discussed and particular attention is devoted to the description of the action of several psychoactive drugs, used currently, including the personal experiences of the authors with adrenochrome, a substance of great importance discovered by the authors.

The excellent biological survey emphasizes quite clearly that man is a multi determined being existing in a complex of interrelations and that biology is one comprehensive basic science in which all aspects of living things blend. The person must be considered as a biological unity, the product of numerous and complex factors, including the historical, the genetic, and prebirth influences, the family life and formal education, social circumstances, and cultural traditions. These are blended into a true integration, that is, into something reactively different from any of the ingredients that compose it.

This being true, in order to get at the pathology of behavior we must not only study the individual in action, but also the brain and the other organs of the body, particularly those that support the brain directly, and finally the whole individual. We should not yield to a modern trend to explain everything in psychodynamic terms, which may seem fairly satisfactory to us, or even help the patient to adjust to the world, to some extent, but we should continue to seek correlations in the physiological and structural parts as well as in the psychological. Although we can, as yet, approach a human being only vectively our attitude should remain holistically oriented, at all times. It may help to remember that we are always in an "organic" state from conception to final complete disintegration.

In the section on therapy, one finds detailed instructions for a total attack on the disorder, directed throughout to the patient and his relatives, with a comprehensive discussion of the pharmacological approaches, including an informative presentation of the nicotinic acid therapy as originated and applied by the authors in their research and practice. Concerning pharmacological studies, there are results that are worth mentioning, in support of the interest in this field. To enumerate just a few of the important achievements of psychoneuropharmacology that have appeared during the past 15 years, one may mention (1) contributions to the knowledge of the structure-function of brain cells as well as of other body cells; (2) demonstration of a biochemical individuality of the brain and the providing of methods for the study of a chemical basis of learning; (3) emphasis on the dependence of some of the pharmacological responses on the situational and social settings; (4) renewal of interest in the placebo response for careful scrutiny, testing and evaluation; (5) indications that the so-called drug-produced experimental "model psychoses" are in some way linked to enzyme systems in the brain; and (6) certain impressions running through the results of published biochemical research showing similarities sufficient to suggest that a chemical factor or factors are involved in schizophrenia. It would seem to be established that there is something different circulating in the blood of schizophrenics than in that of other people. The contributions of the authors of this book have been extensive and outstanding in several of the areas included in the term "psychoneuropharmacology."

Their comments on prevention of schizophrenia deny the validity of the current ideas concerning the causes of schizophrenia ascribed to stress, poverty, disrupted family situations and unequal love for siblings. Such matters apparently have little to do with cause, correction, or prevention of schizophrenia. Moreover, psychotherapy of schizoid children is not indicated as it seems to be useless as a preventive measure. The program as outlined for action is one in which both the ill and members of their families can participate in the understanding and management of the life of the affected person. After evaluating the text as a whole, one becomes convinced that it is the most comprehensive book of the kind yet written.

Although much additional research will be required to fill the gaps still remaining in our knowledge of mental disorders, we have the right to be encouraged with what has been accomplished, when we consider the distance covered during the last 160 years: it was about that long ago that the famous philosopher, Kant, insisted that the subject of mental disorders belonged to philosophy and not to the physician.

Nolen D. C. Lewis, M.D.

AUTHORS' PREFACE

FOR the past seventeen years orthomolecular treatment has become more sophisticated and thus much more effective. The indications for using this therapy are sharper and more widespread. One of the roots of orthomolecular therapy was the use of high doses of vitamin B-3 for treating the schizophrenias. Another was Linus Pauling's investigations and conclusions into molecular medicine culminating with his classic paper in *Science* in 1968. As the treatment has become more scientific, so have the results of treatment vastly improved. This will be described in this revised edition. Unfortunately the vast majority of patients have been denied the benefits of this treatment because psychiatrists still remain willfully ignorant of it, or they might have heard something about it but have accepted the word of the American Psychiatric Association that there is nothing to it, that if a few patients recover it must be a placebo response or else they were not really schizophrenic to begin with. They have denied themselves the pleasure of seeing patients become well but even worse have denied their patients their chance for recovery by the best possible current treatment. There are many explanations for this but no valid excuse. A few days ago I chaired a meeting of the Canadian Schizophrenia Foundation in Toronto. It was held on the main floor of the Clarke Institute, in their auditorium which we rented, but it was not sponsored by the Clarke Institute. They knew the meeting was being held but not a single psychiatrist from their massive staff registered for the meeting, perhaps because it was on a Saturday and they could not be bothered to give up their weekend. They missed a striking panel put on by a psychiatrist who introduced three of her patients all of whom had recovered from their schizophrenia after they had failed to respond to the best modern treatment to which they had been exposed. These patients freely described their hallucinations and delusions which were not ameliorated by the drugs. After they were started on orthomolecular treatment they recovered. Had the psychiatrists allowed themselves the opportunity to attend this meeting they would have seen something they now rarely see, recovered patients able to function normally in our society.

Psychiatrists are fearful of censure from their colleagues and by their licensing boards. If they are academic they are fearful they will forfeit their chance for advancement. A few physicians have lost their license to practice and many more have been threatened with this loss unless they changed their errant ways.

Public pressure will in time remove this fear as has already occurred in Alaska and in Washington State where it is now illegal for licensing boards to penalize their members for practicing with orthomolecular or alternate methods unless they have harmed their patients. The chances of harming a patient by orthomolecular methods is very much less than the chance they will be harmed by the use of powerful xenobiotics, drugs.

ACKNOWLEDGMENTS

THIS book is the joint creation of three authors, Mrs. F. H. Kahan and the two listed on the cover. We wish to acknowledge the fact that without the help of Mrs. Kahan this book would not have been written. It was done as follows—(1) one of us (A.H.) wrote the first draft. In it no attention was given to composition, style and form, but the essential ideas the two of us had discussed for over ten years were assembled. (2) This material was sent to Mrs. Kahan who was asked to rewrite the material into simple language and to remove, as far as possible, any jargon and professional construction. (3) It was then returned to A.H. and a copy sent to H.O. (4) H.O. reviewed it very carefully, made many deletions and additions until he was certain our joint ideas were presented fairly and accurately. (5) It again came to A.H. who once more reviewed the manuscript. (6) It was then returned to Mrs. Kahan and many discussions were held with her. (7) Mrs. Kahan's final manuscript was returned to A.H. who once more edited the manuscript. This was the final one submitted to our good friend, Dr. D. Johnson. Since then we have been guided by his advice and this has improved our manuscript considerably.

We take complete responsibility for the scientific accuracy of the material herein, but we again acknowledge that the credit for the excellent manner in which our ideas are presented belongs to Mrs. F. H. Kahan.

A. HOFFER
H. OSMOND

HOW TO LIVE
WITH
SCHIZOPHRENIA

CHAPTER I

SO YOU HAVE SCHIZOPHRENIA?

So you have schizophrenia. Or you have a relative who has it. Schizophrenia is a long name for a disease which attacks many people all over the world. Babies may be born with it. Small children may get it. Adults of all walks of life and of all ages may have it.

You may find schizophrenics in your school. Or in your lawyer's office. Or in the barber shop. You may have coffee with a schizophrenic every morning. You are rubbing elbows with them every day.

You may have heard of schizophrenia as a frightful mental illness with mysterious effects which must be spoken about in whispers. In fact, years ago schizophrenia was such a bad word that psychiatrists preferred to diagnose a schizophrenic as an immature personality, a depressive or a neurotic to spare the family the terrors it evoked. Even today many psychiatrists hesitate to use the word in diagnosis for fear of "labelling the patient for the rest of his life."

Schizophrenia actually is a very common disease which affects the whole body, and the only mystery is that many people are still unable to recognize it as such.

It is a disease like any other disease, with causes and treatment. When you have certain symptoms, you go to a doctor expecting that he will examine you and make a diagnosis on the basis of his findings. It is the same thing with schizophrenia.

When you have schizophrenia you are actually physically ill, but the symptoms are both physical and mental for the disease has a specific effect on the brain. You may be fatigued, listless or depressed. Your skin may change to a darker hue, and your skin

1

and muscle tone may not be as good as it once was. Your eyes may have a glazed unnatural look.

You will find the chief changes occurring in the way you see, think, feel and act. You may find that you have trouble judging time or distance. People and objects may change into many different shapes and do strange things, like beds moving up the walls. Things may even feel different to the touch because your nerve endings are so much more sensitive than before.

Sounds may seem louder, and what may be ordinary noise to other people may be deafening to you. The disease may have the effect of producing voices in your head or in your ears, telling you what to do. Because of these changes in seeing, hearing and feeling, you begin to think and act differently.

Some schizophrenics feel that others are plotting against them and take steps to protect themselves. Some believe that they are in positions of high authority and act accordingly. Some feel brittle and believe they will break like glass if they smile or move, and so stay in one position for hours at a time.

These are some of the symptoms of schizophrenia, although every patient has degrees and variations of these, depending to some extent upon his own personality.

Schizophrenia has been with us from the beginning of mankind, and has not changed noticeably through time. Dr. John Conolly, physician to the then Middlesex Lunatic Asylum at Hanwell, lecturing at the Royal College of Physicians in London in 1849, described schizophrenia in part as follows:

"He thinks every familiar countenance changed; he believes that sermons are especially addressed to him; he imagines that he hears voices warning him, or threatening him, or urging him to specific actions. He is sure that the popular authors of the day know all about him and write at him. His senses become disturbed; he sees lights shining in the sky, or appearances in the heavens. Sentences are written there, condemning him forever. He feels heated, and thinks the air is on fire, or that some magnetic influences are exercised over him; what he touches seems impure, and what he eats or drinks tastes of poison. He arms himself, or barricades his room; he cherishes secret plans of escape and distant travel; he suspects that his friends will intercept him, and, full of revenge, meditates their destruction. . . . The countenance grows haggard; the eyes have an unnatural brightness and prominence and the pupil is dilated or contracted. . . ."

The natural recovery rate of schizophrenia has remained unchanged throughout the years. Dr. Conolly noted even then that the natural course of the disease accounted for recovery of fifty per cent of the patients.

There is no greater, and no less, incidence of the disease in the population today than there was 100 years ago. Results of a study made in Massachusetts a century ago, compared with today, show that there has been little change. Recent studies of the disease in large groups of people in New York State suggest that there is a slight increase in occurrence. However, much more research will have to be done.

Similarly, until contrary evidence is produced, we must conclude that the disease is the same in every part of the world. Though there are no complete studies for all regions, so far nothing has been found to prove that there are geographical differences in the disease. The Italian schizophrenic has the same illness as the Russian schizophrenic. The schizophrenic in northern Europe has a counterpart in the schizophrenic in the United States. A Canadian psychiatrist walking into a Greek mental hospital will have no trouble picking out the schizophrenics at first sight.

Of course, there will be some differences in the psychological nature of the illness, depending upon the customs of the area the patient comes from, his tradition and religion, for the schizophrenic incorporates the attitudes and beliefs of his society into his psychological systems.

In Canada he may think the Communists are after him and see Communist plots everywhere. In Russia he may think the imperialist capitalists are after him. The African schizophrenic may think his gods have turned on him. The Canadian schizophrenic may hear radio announcers saying obscene things about him. The native in India, who does not have a radio, may think others are talking about him. The content of his delusion may be different, but the delusion of the schizophrenic everywhere may be of the same basic nature.

Before we can understand schizophrenia for what it is, we must take a look at some of the myths that have grown up around it, obscuring it and compounding its tragedies.

One of medicine's proudest achievements today is the refinement of diagnosis and specificity of treatment. For example, at one time fevers were looked upon as being vague and unspecific diseases in themselves, with no relationship to any physical ailments. They were even thought to be related to environmental factors, and were called swamp fever as related to humidity, heat fever and so on.

The first major advance was the thermometer which made it possible to define the severity of fevers and their rhythm over a period of days, weeks, months and even years.

The second major advance was bacteriology, the discovery of disease-producing agents, and later serology, the study of anti-bodies in blood serum when blood samples are taken. Now fever is no longer considered a diagnosis, but a symptom, and when anyone has a fever the doctor looks for specific diseases such as measles, smallpox and pneumonia.

These techniques have enabled us to check many serious diseases. Yet, while medicine continues to make important advances, some psychiatrists prefer to labor Myth No. 1, that diagnosis of schizophrenia is not important and that it is necessary to concentrate only on personality.

This is a backward step which takes us back several centuries to the time when fever was believed to be an illness and not a symptom. It is an anti-scientific movement, and if it gathers much momentum, it will practically stifle any further useful research. It is a prescription for standing still, and instead of the psychiatrists controlling the disease, the disease will continue to control the psychiatrists, like the tail wagging the dog instead of the dog wagging the tail.

Myth No. 2 is that schizophrenia is caused by something being wrong in the personality. Many diseases went through this stage at one time, including general paresis of the insane. Fortunately medicine brought them into proper focus before they ran rampant over our society. The history of general paresis of the insane, a fatal disease resulting from the progressive effect of syphilis, resembles that of schizophrenia in that at one time it was thought to be due to moral, rather than physical, causes.

Dr. Conolly in his lectures over 100 years ago referred to 146 cases of general paralysis in men, all of which ended in death. The causes, he stated, were "ascertained with tolerable certainty in 96 cases." In 60 out of the 96, the disease was ascribed to moral causes, such as "losses, anxiety, grief, domestic unhappiness, disappointments, poverty, reverses, etc." Intemperance, singly, was assigned as a cause in twenty cases only; but in fifteen other cases of the sixty just mentioned, as a cause in combination with losses, grief, etc. The other causes mentioned, each in one or two cases only, are "fever, injury of the head, hot climate, exposure to wet and cold, hereditary disposition, abuse of mercury, sensual excesses, foul air."

Dr. Conolly, in his own private practice, ascribed a large majority of his cases to "moral causes, to some over-exertion, or to some mental shock." He even thought some cases might be due to a severe fall followed by a temporary loss of consciousness. This, as in schizophrenia, is a glorious example of putting the cart before the horse.

Myth No. 3 is that schizophrenia is due to bad mothering. It is remarkable how well established this is in spite of the fact that no research has ever been done which proves it. Many mothers today are suffering needless feelings of guilt because their children's illnesses are related to too early or too harsh toilet training, or quarreling at the breakfast table, or inconsistent discipline, or other irrelevant factors in their histories.

Until now, this was a moderately safe theory because it was difficult to prove wrong. But the only ones to benefit from it were the novelists, because it provided many an idea for a plot. For, after all, can you think of anything more dramatic than a child ending up hopelessly ill in a mental hospital because of his mother?

If the mother is not to blame, the myth goes on, then it must be the father, the husband or the wife. This can be, and is, extended to anything blamable in the family background—poverty, wealth, intemperance, lack of discipline, too much discipline, and other extremities of any kind. So far no one has blamed sons and daughters for their parents' schizophrenia. But parents may have senile psychoses, and the day may come when their children are blamed for that. It is dangerous these days to be the relative of a mentally ill person, for you will probably be blamed for driving him mad.

This scapegoat principle as used by psychiatrists works well in circumventing the necessity for therapists to blame themselves. But it harms not only one individual—the patient whose disease goes on untreated—but two or more individuals, the patient and a loved one or loved ones.

There are many instances of couples advised to divorce

because, for example, the wife is said to be bad for her husband's schizophrenia.

Mr. W., a businessman, and his son Peter are examples of how this theory works when a child fails to respond to psychoanalytic treatment. At the age of four or five Peter began having violent rages and would remain in his room for hours, refusing to talk to anyone. He preferred to play by himself most of the time and was extremely quiet. The alarmed father took him to a clinic where, he was told, it would be necessary to "break through the barriers" to discover what Peter's real underlying conflicts were before treatment could begin.

Several months later, the father took him in desperation to another clinic where play therapy was attempted "to find out why Peter reacted as he did to reality." The third clinic attempted hours of interviews with Peter and his parents, with no noticeable effect on Peter. After wandering with his child from one clinic to another, the father was finally told Peter could not recover because of the father's own attitude.

Grief and guilt began to prey on Mr. W. The professionals to whom he had gone for help had put him on trial, sat in judgment on him and pronounced him guilty. In his own defence he reminded himself that he had helped raise five normal children. But hadn't he also played a major role in the illness of his sixth child, condemning him by his own attitudes to a lifetime of insanity? He brooded about this until he went into serious depression which might have ended in suicide had not an understanding friend helped him pull out of it.

This principle of blaming parents can be called the "time bomb" or "delayed action bomb" principle. It goes something like this: The child suffers trauma as an infant because of something the mother or father has done, and the ego is damaged. For years nothing happens, but one day the trauma suddenly exerts its malicious effect and the child becomes mentally ill.

No other diseases in medicine are known to do this. When you are exposed to measles, for example, you may become ill in a predictable number of days or weeks. Usually, after damage is done to the body, there is a period of repair and the patient gets well. No further damage is done until the illness reappears. (This must not be confused with normal wear and tear in joints, muscles, etc.)

Some psychiatrists, however, prefer to carve a special place for themselves in medical history by fashioning diseases to suit themselves. The disease illogically occurs X years after the seeds have been planted, and repair, we are told, occurs only with psychoanalysis since the trouble lies in a personality defect. The latter is the most pernicious myth of all, for it hinders any attempt to view man's most serious and damaging illness realistically and control it adequately.

It is a pessimistic myth for, if one is ill as a result of something that happened at the age of two, one is doomed forever, because it is impossible to change the past. It is a destructive myth, for it assumes weakness, in the patient or his background, and society has its own inimitable ways of punishing weakness, with prejudice, contempt, indifference, perhaps even imprisonment and execution.

Psychiatrists can point at any one of a number of persons on whom to blame their patients' illnesses and failure to respond to treatment. But the schizophrenic remains maltreated, maligned and misrepresented to the point where his chances of improvement are no better today than they were 100 years ago. In other words, if he does not improve in the natural course of the disease, as fifty per cent of the schizophrenics do, he does not improve at all.

Myth No. 4 is a very modern invention popularized by Dr. R. D. Laing, who considers schizophrenia a search for enlightenment, and by T. Szasz, who claims there is no such thing as mental disease and therefore there is no such disease as schizophrenia. These eccentric views are not based upon serious scientific data. In fact, they are not taken very seriously by these two psychiatrists themselves, since so far they continue to *treat* them as physicians would. If they were serious, they would burn their medical certificates in front of the medical school which erred so grievously in giving them to them, would no longer use their M.D.s and all the privileges associated with them, and would on the one hand be friends and advisors to strange non-patients who need help in their self-search for enlightenment and on the other hand defend the right of these people to suffer the sanctions of society for any of their bizarre behavior if it were illegal.

For these and other reasons, it has been thought necessary to produce a book of this kind, which gives information to patients and their families and which helps them to help themselves.

Unfortunately, families are being given hypotheses, for which there is little or no evidence, as facts. It is our purpose to correct popular misconceptions planted and nurtured by psychiatrists, broadcast by journalists and novelists, in order that we can take logical and practical steps to eliminate schizophrenia as a dread disease, as once we tackled tuberculosis.

Patients are given no information about their illness, neither its cause nor diagnosis. It may seem unimportant to know the name of one's illness. But in our culture, what is unnamed is usually feared.

Of course, some names are more feared than others, but public education can teach people that there is nothing to fear in names themselves. Tuberculosis was once feared, for the same illogical reasons we now fear schizophrenia.

When patients are denied a name for their illness they are denied a very important and necessary role in our society. People who are ill often develop deviant, or different, behavior. Deviant behavior cannot be tolerated by any society since its very basis may be threatened. The role of being sick, therefore, is one of man's most humane inventions, for it allows people their deviant behavior because of illness. Society will not tolerate "badness" but will tolerate the eccentricities of the sick because someone has said they are sick and has given their illness a name.

It is possible the medical profession originated from a profession which confined itself solely to deciding whether deviant behavior in members of the tribe was due to sickness or to some other cause, e.g. badness (to be punished) or possession (to be exorcised).

Thus, a man with a broken leg is not allowed to work, and is given the right to rest, complain and do many things which would be entirely unacceptable if his leg were not broken. Now imagine what position the mental patient is in when he finds himself in a strange world in the hospital, and when his nurses and doctors refuse to tell him what his disease is, and so refuse to give him the sick role. One of the most therapeutic measures known to man is denied him, for if he has an unnamed disease he has no disease.

It is a common practice to conceal the illness in a prettier package, such as nervous breakdown, or emotional disease, but this is even worse for these euphemisms fill the patient with guilt. They allow him to think his problems derive from some defect in personality or some defect in his relationship to his parents which he is completely helpless to alter, and so in effect are blaming the patient for his own illness. In that case why not tell the patient to pull up his socks, take a hard look at his problems and resolve to adopt new attitudes to his own situation?

Harvey, an 11-year-old son of wealthy parents, was considered to be the neighborhood bad boy. He had failed in school, threw temper tantrums in the classroom, bullied smaller children, broken neighbors' windows and generally was looked upon as a disturbing factor in the community.

Harvey became associated with "badness" and just the sight of him was enough to arouse tension in his teachers, classmates and other parents.

Harvey was also probably the most punished pupil in school. By the time he was in grade four the teachers had stopped even trying to "understand" him. Sarcasm, humiliation, corporal punishment dogged his footsteps. Harvey, to the astonishment of his classmates, seemed to rise magnificently above all that with more daring adventures, more temper tantrums accompanied by violent destructive activity, and uncontrollable crying fits in class.

Neighbors kept a wary eye on him and no one had a pleasant word for him until he was finally taken to a psychiatrist who said he was acting in response to an illness which had a name.

The attitude toward Harvey in school, at home and in the neighborhood changed completely. When he cried in furious frustration over his inability to solve an arithmetic problem, the teacher instead of resorting to sarcasm spent an extra few minutes with him until he understood it.

When he misbehaved, she no longer reacted as though he were just "trying to get attention," but helped him over his difficult periods, which gradually became less and less frequent. The neighbors were still wary of him, but substituted friendliness for cold rejection. Harvey, when given a name for his illness, assumed a new and important role in his society. He is sick, and is allowed his bizarre actions because it is known that he is sick.

The reverse process is familiar to most mothers. When your child has a high fever, you allow him his crankiness, his insatiable demands and his peevishness. You can tolerate this because you know it is only temporary and that there is a reason for it. You know the doctor is on his way and that he will leave a prescription which, in a matter of days, will have the disease under control. This tolerance of the child's difficult behavior disappears when the doctor has pronounced him well. Instead of being "sick, poor thing," he is suddenly "spoiled or bad."

What must parents of schizophrenic children feel when they have no such assurance of competent help or early termination of the disease, or when too often they are not told what causes their children to behave as they do?

We have seen the look of relief on many of our patients when we gave them the name of their illness. There was an immediate sense of relaxation. Their parents became relaxed, lost their hostility, and were able to tolerate behavior in their children which was previously unacceptable to them.

This, then, is a book for patients and their relatives. It is meant to be read by them and to serve as a guide to self-help. It proposes to describe schizophrenia in recognizable language, and discuss current theories of the causes of schizophrenia, using the most recent data. Since this is not a textbook, there will be no detailed reference to literature.

It will outline our biochemical psychosocial theory of schizophrenia, and current psychiatric treatments with reference to chemical, psychological and other treatments.

It will discuss preventive psychiatry.

It will, finally, outline a program of action in which both the sick and their parents, brothers, sisters and relatives can take part.

In 1992 myths 3 and 4 have been relegated to the dust bin of history. These myths have caused untold misery and harm and we are fortunate that psychiatry has become enlightened. But there are still a few psychiatrists who cling tenaciously to these beliefs. Within the past few months a patient told me she was told by her psychiatrist that her mother had made her sick. These psychiatrists are the fossils of our profession. For this reason we have allowed these myths to remain in this chapter.

CHAPTER II

WHAT IS SCHIZOPHRENIA?

MANY of the current ideas about schizophrenia are wrong. Even the name is wrong. The term schizophrenia implies that something is divided or split. But the personality is not split into two or three separate personalities as in *The Three Faces of Eve*. There is, in fact, no split whatsoever.

The originator of the term, Eugen Bleuler, referred to a lack of connection between the thinking and the feeling of the patient. Many patients who have been sick for a long time appear to others to have a feeling tone or mood which is not appropriate to what they are talking about. For example, a patient may be crying while relating a humorous incident. Even this splitting, however, is quite rare, and will become rarer still as early treatment becomes generally available.

The meaning of schizophrenia as popularly used by journalists and writers is also wrong. The adjective "schizophrenic" is becoming a part of our language to mean separateness, as in "schizophrenic nation," "schizophrenic attitudes," "schizophrenic politics." As used in this way it may impart some vague meaning to the reader, but it actually has no meaning in relation to the disease from which it comes.

An older term, *dementia praecox*, the precocious or parboiled madness, meant that patients early in life became mentally incapacitated. This concept, useful sixty years ago, is no longer correct or useful.

The word "schizophrenia," therefore, serves no useful purpose either in referring accurately to a symptom or a disease, and will some day be replaced by more suitable diagnostic terms, just as "fevers" was replaced as a diagnosis by definite diseases.

Schizophrenia does not, as some claim, have a special affinity for the poor. It is a disease which is prevalent in all cultures and societies and is, as far as we can tell, fairly evenly distributed among all races of men, no matter where they are. It is found as often among Africans and Europeans as among Eskimos and Asians.

Even the most enthusiastic supporters of the theory that schizophrenia is related to poverty have been able to produce only one study to support their claim, where it was found that there were twice as many schizophrenics among the poor. But since about one per cent of a population will have schizophrenia in their lifetime, this is not a particularly remarkable finding and probably was due to many other factors which were not adequately studied.

Other investigators have not found any evidence to show that poverty breeds schizophrenia. The evidence instead is fairly clear that patients who do not recover from schizophrenia tend to drift downward to a standard of living below that of their fathers who do not have the disease. The reason for this is simply that the patients are unable to continue in their work or function effectively in their society. In striking contrast, neurotic patients may remain the same, drift below or climb above their parents' social station.

Schizophrenia and Stress

Schizophrenia, in spite of popular belief, seems to have hardly anything to do with stress. Just as it occurs uniformly among all classes of men, so has it remained unchanged throughout the years, as unconcerned about man's varying fortunes as about the color of his skin and his religion.

Other diseases show remarkable fluctuations through history. Before sanitation was widely practised, epidemics of various diseases would sweep across the population and decimate man. Malnutrition followed the seasons. During the war starvation and disease were rampant.

Diseases due to bacteria, nutritional deficiencies, etc., have shown major swings in prevalence and incidence, and once this was understood simple measures were employed to reduce them drastically.

Chlorinating water destroyed typhoid and other diseases.

Immunization eradicated smallpox and diphtheria, and polio vaccine promises to do the same for polio. Adding nicotinamide to flour in North America has practically eradicated pellagra.

It can be said, in fact, that the first large-scale program of preventive psychiatry was begun, not by psychiatrists nor by psychologists, but by nutritionists. At one time nearly ten per cent of the patients admitted to some mental hospitals in the southern states of America had a disease called pellagra, caused by a lack of a vitamin. The psychological symptoms of this disease resemble schizophrenia so closely that it is likely that many more patients admitted as schizophrenics actually had pellagra. When nutritionists persuaded the United States government to add nicotinic acid to the flour consumed by its citizens, there was a major decrease in this disease. But schizophrenia has remained remarkably unchanged. During war or peace, in periods of poverty or prosperity, it has continued to take its toll in a steady relentless manner.

Its constancy through good times or bad strongly suggests that stress has no relation to schizophrenia. But even this is not conclusive, for no one seems to know for sure what stress really is. Many articles in popular journals picture modern society as being particularly stressful due to its complexities. There is remarkably little evidence, however, that communities today are suffering more stress than those of 100 or even 1,000 years ago.

Primitive man, fondly believed to have been healthy, contented, and wise, was actually according to medical history diseased, discontented and ignorant. Perhaps that is why he had to seek refuge in religion and philosophy.

One needs only to read the novels of the mid-19th century to learn that our ancestors lived constantly with death, filth, privation, fear and pain. A large proportion of women died miserably in childbirth and a large proportion of men, worn out by struggle, died by the time they were fifty. No family was free of death. In fact, if pain and discomfort are some factors which cause stress, then our century by all standards must enjoy less stress than any other. Few can deny that modern societies are characterized by less pain, less illness and greater comfort than ever before.

All we can say for sure, then, is that if stress, whatever it is, does play a role in causing schizophrenia, it is not an important one.

Stress, however, does play a role, as it does with any disease.

The normal stresses which usually cause little difficulty are very real problems to the schizophrenic. In the same way that walking is not stressful to a normal person, to a man with a broken leg it is very stressful indeed. One should expect a schizophrenic to have difficulty. He should be therefore shielded from severe stress when ill and convalescing and supported as much as possible. However, there is no recovery until any and every stress is dealt with in a normal way.

Stress and the Sex Factor

Stress also fails to explain the sex factor in this disease. It is estimated that its incidence among boys below the age of 13 is three to seven times higher than among girls the same age. If the stress theory is correct, one would have to assume that little boys are given three to seven times as much stress as little girls. Dr. F. Kallman has challenged psychodynamic psychiatrists to lower the incidence of schizophrenia in children by persuading parents to be as kind to their sons as they are to their daughters.

Between puberty and the mid-thirties, the incidence is about the same for both boys and girls. Stress theorists would now have to assume that stress on females had increased remarkably after the age of puberty to raise their incidence to equal that of boys.

Death is one of the best ways of assessing stress, and Hans Selye has defined stress in animals as a proportional death rate. Yet from the menopause onward, and at a time in life when men die more frequently than women, more women become schizophrenic than men. So that during a life period when stress is apparently greater in men, as indicated by the higher death rate, they develop schizophrenia less frequently than women.

Is Schizophrenia Inherited?

The final death blow to stress theories, however, has been dealt by studies of twins. There are two kinds of twins, those who come from two separate eggs separately conceived by different sperms, and those who come from one fertilized egg which by some chance divides, each part producing one whole individual.

Twins of the first kind are no more related than if they were ordinary brothers and sisters, and one may be a boy and the other a girl. These are called fraternal twins. The other twins, called identical twins, are so much alike in form and structure that it is often difficult to tell one from the other, and they must be of the same sex. They have nearly identical genetic factors and are as much alike as it is possible to be.

If inheritance plays a major role in schizophrenia, then the chances of one identical twin developing schizophrenia if the other has it, should be much higher than among fraternal twins. This has, in fact, been shown to be the case in excellent studies in the United States and in Europe. If one member of a set of identical twins becomes a schizophrenic, the other has an 85 per cent chance of becoming schizophrenic, even though the twins may be separated at birth and raised in different homes by different parents.

In sharp contrast, the concordance drops among fraternal or two-egg twins to the level of brothers and sisters who are not twins, which is about 15 per cent. These facts have been established beyond doubt, although some psychiatrists who use a double standard of reasoning (a very rigid criterion for biological factors and a very loose set of criteria for psychological factors) seem strangely unaware of these striking differences.

It is thus quite clear that schizophrenia can be determined by one's genes, but there is no simple or direct inheritance, as for eye color. There are a number of genes involved and one can only say what could probably occur in a family.

The majority of schizophrenic patients come from normal parents. But for schizophrenics and their families who may wonder what their chances are of passing on schizophrenia-bearing genes, the following are reasonable estimates of the probabilities:

One-sixth of the children who have a schizophrenic mother or father will have enough genes to make them schizophrenic. That is, out of 100 children who each have one schizophrenic parent, 17 will get it. If both parents are schizophrenic, the proportion is increased to 60 out of 100.

If a brother or sister is schizophrenic, another brother or sister has a 15 per cent chance of having it also. This does not mean that patients with schizophrenia should not have children. It is obvious, too, that sterilizing all schizophrenics would have very little effect in reducing the number of patients and should not be considered. The disease has shown a high-survival value throughout the centuries in spite of the fact that many schizophrenics have no interest in sex and many others were, until ten years ago, kept isolated inside mental hospitals. Today, thanks to new drugs, more schizophrenics are able to live in the community than ever before and we predict that the disease will, over a period of many years, affect many more people.

The New York Times, March 1, 1964, carried the following story:

"Births Widening Type of Insanity"
Rise in Schizophrenic Rate
Called Alarming in State

Professor Franz Kallman reported:

A large-scale study in New York State mental hospitals has shown that within two decades the reproductive rates of schizophrenic women increased 86 per cent, compared with an increase of 25 per cent by the general population.

Dr. Kallman warned that this rise, reflecting the difference between early handling of schizophrenic patients and modern treatment methods, might result in a steady increase of the serious mental disorder. He predicted that the birth-rate among schizophrenics might eventually surpass that of the general population.

We do not know whether the prevalence of schizophrenia should be suppressed, even if it could be. It is possible it is one of the evolutionary experiments not yet under control, and there is not enough evidence today to interfere with that great force in life. There is, however, a lot of evidence to indicate that in many ways people with schizophrenia who have been cured, are healthier physically and mentally than their non-schizophrenic brethren. Schizophrenics appear more youthful, their skin does not crinkle as quickly, their hair retains its pigment longer and the fat under their skin seems to last better. They have fewer allergies, can stand pain much better, and do not get medical shock as easily.

It may be, then, that if the evolutionary experiment works well, everyone will some day have enough of the desirable schizophrenic genes to make them more fit.

Parents who have schizophrenia, however, should learn what

they can about it, and if it should occur in one of their children, seek immediate appropriate help. We hope that they will be able to do this more effectively after having read this book. Families which seem to have more than the expected number of schizophrenics should seek help early whenever one of them shows any sign of illness or of peculiar behavior.

Physical Changes—Undesirable

What, then, is schizophrenia? How can we tell when it is present?

There are physical as well as psychological changes in schizophrenia, some of which are desirable. In general, the earlier the disease strikes the more severely it affects the body. If children become ill before their sensory organs reach full functional maturity, they may never develop normally. The organs themselves may be physically healthy, but their function and coordination may be distorted.

It is possible for skilled child psychiatrists to diagnose schizophrenia at the age of one month by the complete lack of muscle tone. Mothers who have had normal babies notice the queer feeling that, when picked up, their schizophrenic infants sag like limp dolls.

When schizophrenia occurs before puberty, the patients may be smaller in stature than non-schizophrenics, and often are narrow in the chest from front to back. When the left side is compared with the right side, there is found to be a deformity in shape.

When the disease strikes adults, many things can happen. Both men and women are then more susceptible to tuberculosis and are more likely to develop an infection if exposed to this disease. It is quite clear that tuberculotic lesions also heal more slowly in schizophrenics. This was an important cause of death in mental hospitals before they introduced modern methods of tuberculosis control. However, when modern control measures and proper treatments are used, the incidence of tuberculosis among schizophrenics is reduced, but not to normal levels

It is not true that tuberculosis patients are more susceptible to schizophrenia. This proves that the sequence of events is very important, and it will be discussed later.

Another important change is the pronounced fatigue and listlessness which descends upon the patient. This occurs in all physical illnesses and is not peculiar to schizophrenia. The patient usually feels less tired in the morning after sleep, but becomes progressively more and more tired as the day goes on. Toward evening he is often much more psychotic.

Schizophrenic men may become impotent and show atrophy of the male gonads. Women may suffer changes in the menstrual cycle but this returns to normal if the disease vanishes. Both men and women tend to suffer a decrease in sex interest. Schizophrenic men occasionally become confused in their sex identity, possibly due to bizarre feelings. This led Freud to the erroneous belief that repressed homosexuality is at the root of all paranoid ideas. The vast majority of researches designed to test this point have shown that Freud's hypothesis is wrong.

Physical Changes—Desirable

There are a number of tests which show that schizophrenic body fluids differ from those of normal people and those with other psychiatric illnesses. Schizophrenics as a result have desirable physical attributes which non-schizophrenics may well envy.

Schizophrenics are frequently very attractive physically. They tend to age and lose their hair color more slowly, and generally appear more youthful than their chronological age.

They are, furthermore, much freer of many of the physical complaints of man, and seem to be able to survive misfortunes which would kill other people.

Dr. John Lucy found that schizophrenics can take enormous quantities of histamines, the chemical substance which is responsible for allergies in some people. This resistance to histamine explains why allergies are rare among them. A. J. Lea, in a careful study, found one allergic condition in 500 schizophrenics. Other investigators have made similar findings. This is a characteristic of the disease itself and not the patient, for patients can and do develop allergies when they are free of schizophrenia. D. H. Funkenstein reported in 1960 on a group of psychotic patients who had asthma when they were not suffering from schizophrenia, but never had the two together. Rheumatoid arthritis is also very rare in schizophrenia. Thus Dr. D. Gregg reported in *The American Journal of Psychiatry* in 1939 that, out of 3000 autopsies on patients with psychosis, who died for other reasons, not one patient had any evidence of arthritis in their joints or bones. Doctors Nissen and Spencer found no cases of arthritis among 2200 psychotic subjects and Doctors Trevethen and Tatum in 1954 in examining 9000 admissions to a general hospital, 80 had arthritis but not one had schizophrenia.

It has also been noted in mental hospitals that *diabetes mellitus* is an unusual occurrence. Both mental hospitals in Saskatchewan, with a total population of over 3000, have less than five diabetics. Dynamic psychiatrists have explained this by saying that patients who have one "defence mechanism," schizophrenia, have no need for another, diabetes. They have not yet explained in what way diabetes is a defence mechanism any more than they have explained schizophrenia as having a stress basis. It is interesting to note, however, that doctors continue to treat diabetes with insulin and not with psychotherapy.

Schizophrenics can suffer extensive burns, severe injuries, fractures and heart attacks, acute appendicitis and even self-mutilation with abnormal stoicism and detachment. While some people faint when blood is drawn, one schizophrenic patient cut his throat and bled so much that he required five pints of blood, with little sign of shock. Some have cut off fingers and hands without collapsing or appearing to be affected in any other way. They have been known to escape shock symptoms usually suffered at the beginning of a perforated ulcer. ·

Some, of course, do go into deep shock and die, but others seem to benefit from shock when it does occur. One patient, a chronic schizophrenic with bizarre ideas and behavior, suffered very severe burns over a large portion of her body in a kitchen accident. She went into deep traumatic shock, and after a lengthy period of recovery, emerged completely clear mentally and able to return to her family.

This resistance to pain can be dangerous, for acute illnesses are often ignored until too late. Psychotic patients die more often from ruptured hearts than normals, without complaining of pain or giving other signs of severe difficulty.

In 1964 Sir Julian Huxley, Professor E. Mayr and the two of us suggested that the biological advantages present in some schizophrenics accounted for the constant rate of prevalence, even though there should have been a gradual decrease in the incidence of the disease. The usual incarceration in hospitals, combined with the decreased fertility of schizophrenic women and decreased sexual drive of many male schizophrenics, should have had this outcome. We suggested that schizophrenia is part of a genetic polymorphism. This means that some non-schizophrenic relatives of schizophrenics have biological advantages over the normal population. Drs. Michael Carter and C. A. H. Watts (*Brit. J. Psychiatry* Vol. *118*, page 453-460, 1971) examined this idea by comparing relatives of schizophrenics with relatives of carefully matched controls. They found a decreased incidence of virus infections among relatives of schizophrenics (but not of bacterial infections), a decrease in accidents, a decrease in allergies, and an increase in fertility. This is evidence that the schizophrenic genes do impart some biological advantage. It is an advantage to have these genes, to have some of the biochemistry of a schizophrenic, but of course not to be ill from schizophrenia.

Psychological Changes

It is impossible to catalogue and describe all the psychological changes which can occur in schizophrenia. Even if one could, it would be of little value, for the diagnosis of schizophrenia does not depend upon the counting of these symptoms.

There is no personality which is peculiar to schizophrenia. There is no particular type of personality preceding it and it does not impose a uniform type of personality on all patients. Schizophrenics represent all personality types. Opponents of biological theories of schizophrenia have used this as an argument, on the assumption that any biological disease would have the effect of making all patients act the same way. This is a novel idea, since it is not true of any disease so far discovered. *Diabetes mellitus* does not produce uniform personalities any more than schizophrenia does, but no one argues that it is not a physical disease.

Only one personality is believed to precede the disease, and it has found its way into the literature as the schizoid personality. A schizoid personality is supposed to resemble schizophrenia and is usually applied to a person who is ingoing, introverted, quiet, and enjoys seclusion. It was believed that children who were shy and quiet by nature were pre-schizophrenic and parents of such children were advised by physicians to be concerned about them. So strong was this assumption that much research money was spent trying to establish that schizophrenics would come largely from that group known as schizoid personalities. One such study was completed in Toronto, where an examination was made of a large number of school children from an upper-class section of society.

Using certain criteria, a small number of schizoid children were selected. Over the next few years it was found that childhood schizophrenia occurred more frequently in children who had not been selected as schizoid. A similar study in the University of Texas, Dallas, yielded similar results. A large group of children seen in a mental health clinic were classed into extroverted, introverted and ambiverted groups. Of these, the introverted ones would most closely resemble the schizoid people. Over a long follow-up period it was found that the introverted group produced less than the expected share of schizophrenic patients. In fact, out of ten subjects found to have been diagnosed schizophrenic, only one was classified introverted. Three were extroverted and six ambiverted. It thus appears that many introverted and retiring people have been needlessly annoyed by this error.

Since it has not been shown that schizoid subjects produce more schizophrenics than any other personality types, where did this idea originate?

It seems likely the idea came from the necessity of taking histories and the habit of mistaking the first signs of the disease for a special personality preceding it. This is another example of putting symptoms before causes, leading to wrong conclusions. It is as scientific as the procedures adopted by the wise men called upon by the king to determine why the wind blows. The wise men studied the problem for a long time without coming up with any satisfactory answers. It was observed, however, that whenever the wind blew the trees waved. It was, therefore, concluded that the trees' waving produced the wind.

The basic personality is altered by the disease. This is not unique for schizophrenia, since it has been known for centuries that any illness alters personality. A subject with a painful headache may have at the time an irritable, withdrawn, seclusive personality which becomes relaxed, friendly, tolerant and outgoing again when the headache disappears.

The confusion on this point may be due to the characteristic way in which the disease begins. Most diseases give definite and unmistakable warning of their presence fairly early in their history. They have obvious physical manifestations which make it relatively simple for others to accept the fact that the patient has now become sick. If there is a personality change with cancer, for instance, it is understood that this is the result of pain and suffering and allowances are made.

But schizophrenia is often treacherous. It may come on so slowly and insidiously that, like watching the hourly hand of a clock, one sees no beginning or end of the movement. There is nothing definable that one can see, like the sudden loss of weight or unusual pallor, or feel, like a sharp pain in the abdomen. It makes its changes gradually where they are least noticeable, in a slowly increasing personality deformation without any obvious explanation.

If one examines the clinical history of many patients, it becomes obvious that there were personality changes which included withdrawal, shyness, etc., long before schizophrenia was fully developed, or recognized. Perhaps this is why personality theorists have fallen into the trap of believing there is a personality which is predisposed toward it. In these cases, however, the so-called schizoid personality was the first sign that schizophrenia was present, and was a symptom and not a predisposing factor. The term "schizoid," then, has no clinical value and might well be dropped from usage.

Warning Signs

Since the personality of patients with schizophrenia differs as widely as the personality of subjects who do not have this disease, the psychological tests used to measure personality in diagnosis of schizophrenia have no value.

Many clinical psychologists favor Rorschach and other projective tests designed to determine whether we are fun-loving party-goers or sinister types harboring malice and ill-will toward our fathers. These tests have been useless in either diagnosing or helping to treat schizophrenia.

The Rorschach test was developed by Herman Rorschach about forty years ago. It consists of a set of ten cards, with a symmetrical ink blot on each card. The blot is usually black, but is sometimes red. The subject is supposed to look at it and tell the tester of what it reminds him.

What the patient says is interpreted by psychologists who have spent many months memorizing the significance of these comments and who have their own individual ways of analysing the results.

The theory of this kind of tests is that the blots act as a kind of magnet pulling clues to his basic problems from the subject's subconscious. These are supposed to provide the key to personality and diagnosis. Attempts to show that the Rorschach has some value have been singularly unsuccessful, but its use goes on and on.

There is one important unchanging characteristic of the disease to look for, and that is alteration in personality. Whenever there is a change in character, without an accompanying clear change in the environment and in the absence of physical illness, one may suspect schizophrenia.

This change is marked by a turning into oneself and an intensification or exaggeration of abnormal and asocial traits. For example, if a normal outgoing adolescent over a period of years becomes shy, seclusive, lonely and irritable, this is a serious personality change and parents should look for the cause. In a proportion of cases, they will find schizophrenia.

Change in personality, then, is the hallmark of schizophrenia. In order to evaluate the change we must know what the personality changed from, and must consider the age at which the change occurred. The easiest patients to diagnose on the basis of change are those who have reached the end of the developing years and have achieved stable personalities.

Schizophrenia is very difficult to diagnose in the first ten years of life. In fact, several decades ago it was believed that schizophrenia did not occur at all under the age of ten. Of course it does, but its diagnosis requires skill. Trained and skillful psychiatrists can even diagnose it at the age of one month, but these experts are extremely rare.

Several years ago a professor from Michigan, R. Rabinovitch, who was in Saskatoon, Saskatchewan, for a conference, remarked on the extremely low incidence of childhood schizophrenia in this province. It occurred, he noted, only one-twentieth as often as in Michigan, an interesting phenomenon in view of the fact that the disease in adulthood occurred so uniformly across all regions. He concluded that its low incidence in Saskatchewan children was due to the fact that there were too few psychiatrists here able to diagnose it. Undoubtedly the majority of schizophrenic children in this province were called behavioral problems or considered to be mentally retarded.

One reason for confusing schizophrenia with retardation in the young is again due to our habit of diagnosing symptoms instead of the disease. Human beings, animals and birds all have critical learning periods in their development. The song-learning period in birds, for example, is about a year. If a young male chaffinch is isolated from others of his kind at the age of three or four days, he doesn't learn the complete chaffinch song. But if he hears an adult bird singing before he learns to sing himself, he will in a year produce the song of his species, whether he is isolated or not. Similarly, there is a ten-day period just after weaning when mice learn to fight. If mice are kept by themselves at twenty days of age, they do not fight as readily in adulthood as those brought up in groups.

There is a critical period in human beings when they learn to speak, and in other ways prepare themselves for the learning which lies ahead. If, for some reason, they are unable to learn during this period, they may not learn at all.

If schizophrenia occurs under the age of ten, it will interfere with the learning process and the child's learning may be permanently impaired. Since we cannot distinguish a clear personality change, therefore, we take note of his failing school grades or his inability to keep up with others of his age. The inevitable diagnosis then is retardation, and the child is forced into the special place reserved in our society for that group of people, from which there seems to be no escape.

Personality in the next ten years of life is better established, but still unsettled. Therefore, schizophrenia becomes easier to diagnose, but the danger is great that the adolescent's illness will take a form which many will confuse with simply "adolescent behavior."

A large proportion of adolescent schizophrenics are called anxiety neuroses, adolescent turmoil or other such terms. When the disease first strikes during the second ten years of life, however, the patient has a better chance of recovery. The main difficulty here is that education is interrupted for several years as the disease develops, and during treatment and convalescence.

It is during maturity that schizophrenia is most readily diagnosed, for at this period of life, personality has more or less stabilized and change in personality can be determined more readily.

The only period during maturity when the diagnosis is easily missed is during the period after women have had their babies, when the illness is frequently mistaken for depression, and during the menopause when most illnesses are called involutional depressions. The final period of life when diagnosis is difficult is when old age or senility develops, for then many mental illnesses are confused with senile psychosis.

How the Changes Come About

Since this book is not a textbook of psychiatry we will describe how these changes in personality come about. These are the psychological changes which occur so frequently in schizophrenics. They will be described under four main headings: (*a*) perception; (*b*) thought; (*c*) mood; (*d*) activity.

Perception—The Way Things Appear to Us

Inside every human being is a finely woven network of nerves which take messages from ear, eye, nose, skin and taste buds to the brain. Here they are worked upon by a vastly complicated system of chemicals, each with certain duties to perform, and various departments charged with the heavy job of advising different parts of the body what to do. There is an instant interpretation, which is telegraphed back to the parts directly concerned, whereupon the individual gets angry, excited, frightened, pleased, or in other ways acts appropriately in response, depending a great deal on his own personality.

This is perception. The five senses provide us with information we must have about our own bodies and the world around us if we are to survive. They pick up cues from other people; the tone of voice, the facial expression, the gestures, and these play an important part in how we get along with them.

In addition to the five senses there are other important senses, and one of these is the passing of time. Another is knowing where your hand is, or relying on your feet to perform certain jobs without any special prodding from you. In other words, in normal individuals perception is spontaneous, automatic and perfectly co-ordinated.

Suppose, however, something interferes with the way messages are taken to the brain and the individual receives a distorted picture. Still acting appropriately to the information received by the brain, he is now acting inappropriately to his situation. His judgement may then be impaired and he cannot think clearly.

Or suppose because of interference with messages in the brain one has to stop and think what one's feet are doing. Suppose when you are reading the words jump up and down, and you are so interested in what the word is doing, you forget to think about what it means.

Suppose you can no longer remember what your mother looks like unless you piece an image of her together, piece by piece, and then have to concentrate to hang on to it. Suppose you hear a voice telling you to go hang yourself. Suppose, because sounds are too loud, you are distracted and can no longer concentrate on the simplest things, like watching TV.

All these things can and do happen in people, and they happen when the person has schizophrenia.

In schizophrenia the world and people in it have changed. Dr. Andrew McGhie and Dr. James Chapman in England have collected descriptions from various schizophrenic patients on how the disease has affected them, and find that disturbance in areas of perception and attention is primary in this disease. Normal conversation is disrupted. "When people are talking," said one patient, "I just get scraps of it. If it is just one person who is speaking that's not so bad, but if others join in, then I can't pick it up at all. I just can't get into tune with that conversation. It makes me feel open, as if things are closing in on me and I have lost control. Movements become slower because each one must be thought out." "People go about completely unthinking,", said another. "They do things automatically. A man can walk down the street and not bother. If he stops to think about it, he might look at his legs and just wonder where he is going to get the energy to move his legs. His legs will start to wobble. How does he know that his legs are going to move when he wants them to?"

Or as another patient put it, "If I do something, like going for a drink of water, I have to go over each detail. Find cup, walk over, turn tap, fill cup, turn tap off, drink it. I keep building up a picture. I have to change the picture each time. I have to make the old picture move. I can't concentrate. I can't hold things. Something else comes in. Various things. It's easier if I stay still."

Schizophrenia can change one or all of our sensory modes, and this produces the bizarre thinking and behavior which is characteristic of the disease.

1. VISUAL CHANGES

The sense of vision is one of the primary senses and is trusted more than most of the others. The statement "seeing is believing" expresses a profound truth. Many changes in perception can occur as follows:

(i) *Changes in Color.* Colors may become very brilliant or, more frequently, lose their brilliance. Sometimes the whole world becomes a uniform monotonous grey. When this happens it is not clear whether the patient sees all colors, but has lost his normal emotional reaction to them, or whether he sees all colors the same. The patient during this period may be unaware the world is different. One patient realized her world had been dull and grey only after she suddenly regained normal color vision.

"Colors seem to be brighter now, almost as if they are luminous," one patient told Dr. Chapman and Dr. McGhie. "When I look around me it's like a luminous painting. I'm not sure if things are solid until I touch them."

Another patient said: "I am noticing colors more than before, although I am not artistically minded. The colors of things seem much more clear and yet, at the same time, there is something missing. The things I look at seem to be flatter as if I were looking just at a surface. Maybe it's because I notice so much more about things and find myself looking at them for a longer time. Not only the color of things fascinates me but all sorts of little things like markings in the surface, pick up my attention, too."

(ii) *Changes in Form.* Objects remain recognizable but look different. This may lead patients to believe the objects are unreal, that is, that they have a new, unexpected and, therefore, unreal quality. Sometimes pictures are seen as having real three-dimensional quality. A house in a picture may appear to have the depth and perspective of a house on the street. On the other hand, three-dimensional objects may appear flat.

Angles may become distorted. Instead of lines going up and down or straight across, they may seem to be leaning over. Sometimes objects develop life-like qualities and pulsate, as though they were breathing. Words on paper may move up and down or sideways, and lines may appear to crowd together. Parallel lines or patterns on wooden objects or in floors may flow in and out as if alive.

(iii) *Misidentification.* The ability to distinguish one face from another depends upon being able to see properly. The slightest change in a face is enough to make it seem strange or different.

One male patient said people's shapes did strange things. Sometimes their faces were triangular or square. Sometimes their heads got larger or smaller. Sometimes one shoulder went up and the other went down. For this reason, he couldn't look at people for very long, but had to look away.

"But you're looking at me now," said the social worker.

"Yes, but you don't bother me," he said. "I'm used to you. In fact, you look rather funny."

If visual perception is disturbed the subject may lose his ability to recognize people. *The New York Herald Tribune* February 12, 1964, carried the following story under the heading, "Killer Says Voices Told Me To Shoot":

> When he came down the stairs he had unnatural feet, iridescent eyes and his fangs were showing. My voices told me to shoot him. Police said A had suffered a nervous breakdown after his father's death.

Clearly what happened was that A was very psychotic and suffering from auditory hallucinations. When poor young Mr. Burke came down the stairs A saw him coming down. Looking up at him could strongly enhance any failures in constancy, since it seems our perceptions are more stable along the horizontal plane.

Another patient had a similar misidentification with serious consequences. During a period of deep depression and anxiety he looked up and saw a young girl coming down the stairs. She seemed to be surrounded by a halo and looked like an angel. This psychotic man immediately fell in love with her. This eventually led to his divorce and to a prolonged period of extreme tension and unhappiness.

An elderly schizophrenic who had been sick for ten years knew she was married to Mr. Jones. But when asked if Mr. Jones was sitting beside her, she was unable to recognize him and denied it.

A male patient lost his ability to tell one face from another. All faces seemed the same to him, leading him to believe he was being followed.

Some patients notice changes in themselves when they look in the mirror and find these disturbing. One patient's chief symptom was that she saw bags and lines under her eyes. None of these were present but she could see them and this had a profound effect upon her. She became quiet and seclusive and refused to go out.

Some patients may also see themselves as being much younger or older than they really are and this leads to problems.

(iv) *Changes in Far Vision Perspective.* A common complaint of schizophrenic patients deals with the ability to orient themselves. Subjects who ride in cars become insecure and feel either that passing cars are coming toward them too closely when they are not, or that they themselves are too close to the ditch. Because of this, several patients stopped driving cars as their illness developed. These visual changes also make it difficult for patients to estimate correctly the size of people and objects far from them. Some see other people much smaller than they really are.

These changes send patients to oculists or ophthalmologists from whom they demand glasses. Most often the new glasses do not solve the problem, and a frequent symptom of schizophrenia, therefore, is a frequent change of glasses with no relief.

A common problem among sufferers from the disease concerns the ability to judge whether people are looking directly at them or not. The ability to decide whether one is being looked at depends upon a proper binocular vision and a very exact coordination of a variety of cues. If the area of the brain which judges convergence is not functioning properly, subjects would be inclined to see people as looking at them when they are not.

In a study involving schizophrenic and non-schizophrenic patients, we found that twenty-five schizophrenic patients were less able to decide whether an investigator was looking into their eyes than a group of thirty non-schizophrenic patients.

The schizophrenic is liable to feel that he is being looked at long and more often than usual, when this is not so. The earliest symptom of schizophrenia may be the inability to lose the feeling of being watched. Recently a professor of biology sought a psychiatric consultation because he was continually and painfully aware that his students were watching him as he lectured to them. He was disturbed that, after many years of lecturing, this feeling was still present and much stronger than it had been. The urine test showed he was very ill with malvaria.

Whether people are looking at us or not, and how they look at us, produces an emotional reaction in most people and would, therefore, have a profound effect on the schizophrenic.

In a letter to Dr. Osmond, Edward T. Hall, Department of Political and Social Science, Illinios Institute of Technology in Chicago, wrote, "I think that the point about the schizophrenic not being able to tell when people are looking at him is very important. Its importance, as a matter of fact, has undoubtedly been overlooked. Recently, I have had my students doing experiments on eye behaviour. . . . One of the first things I discovered was that my own feelings about being looked at in certain ways that often caused me to be quite anxious, were actually shared by a great many people. I had thought that my own discomfort was due to a failure on my part in working through some old dynamism that was buried in my past experience. This may also be so, but the data indicate that the reaction is a normal one and can be exceedingly painful."

He went on to point out that "dominant baboons can cause a younger baboon to scream with pain at a distance of around thirty feet simply by looking at him." He concluded that if the schizophrenic's capacity to tell when people are looking at him is seriously disturbed, he could be in deep difficulties. He also had observed that "they use their eyes in a very improper way" creating hostility or anxiety in those around them.

In ordinary life there is a kind of visual exchange between one person and the other and the eyes are normally used to facilitate social relations. When people talk, they look at each other and look away again. They may look at a person's mouth, shoulder, or the top of his head. They rarely look directly into each other's eyes except for very short intervals, for being stared at makes many people uncomfortable. In fact, small children are often told not to stare.

Many animals are disturbed when they are stared at. A bore can be temporarily halted or completely silenced by gazing straight into his eyes. Freud placed his patients on a couch because he disliked being looked at for hours on end.

The feeling of being watched or stared at, then, would be reason enough for a person to remain in seclusion.

(v) *Illusions and Hallucinations.* Schizophrenics do not, as we are told, "imagine" they hear or see things which are not there. They actually hear and see them. They have illusions because something has gone wrong with the way they perceive things and, therefore, they misinterpret what they are looking at. The coat hanging in a cupboard may momentarily look like a man or a bear.

Hallucinations are things, scenes, people, etc., which patients see but which other people do not see. Visual hallucinations can be anything familiar to everyone in everyday life, or may be fantastic visions of the kind seen during transcendental states or during experiences induced by psychotomimetic drugs like mescalin and LSD-25.

(vi) *General Comments.* Visual changes may range in intensity from very slight to very severe, and may endure from a hallucination of a single moment to hallucinations lasting many decades. The response or reaction of the subject to his visual changes depends upon many things. This will be discussed further on in this book when the comprehensive theory of schizophrenia is considered in Chapter IV.

Some psychiatrists try to distinguish between so-called true and pseudo- (not true) hallucinations. They accept hallucinations to be true when the patient sees any physical familiar object which no one else can see, and believes it to be real. Pseudo-hallucinations are said to be the same visions, but when the patient realizes them to be phantasms or visions.

If this were the only matter at issue, there would be no quarrel with these arbitrary definitions. But psychiatrists have used these distinctions to make diagnosis even more unclear and difficult, for it is now said that schizophrenics have true hallucinations and hysterics have pseudo-hallucinations. If the psychiatrist wishes to give the patient psychotherapy he will be tempted to call them pseudo-hallucinations.

Actually, diagnosis depends not upon the patient and his hallucinations, but upon the psychiatrist. If the latter thinks the patient has hysteria, he terms the hallucinations "pseudo"; if he believes the patient to have schizophrenia, his hallucinations are said to be true. The definition, therefore, is tied to the idea of the diagnosis. It would be scientifically better to drop these terms "true" and "pseudo" and merely say instead that the patient has hallucinations.

2. AUDITORY CHANGES

There can be fewer changes in hearing than in seeing. Sounds may be louder, or not as loud.

"It's as if someone had turned up the volume," one patient said. "I notice it most with background noises—you know what I mean, noises that are always around but you don't usually notice them. Now they seem to be just as loud and sometimes louder than the main noises that are going on. . . . It's a bit alarming at times because it makes it difficult to keep your mind on something when there's so much going on that you can't help listening to."

Sounds may become less intelligible and harder to locate. One patient, for instance, said that though he knew the sounds were coming from the wireless in front of him, they seemed to be coming from behind his back.

Very few schizophrenic patients are free from auditory changes. As a result, textbooks of psychiatry regard auditory hallucinations as a sign of a more serious disease process, while visual hallucinations are taken more lightly. However, the evidence to support these views is not strong, since psychiatrists fail to make careful studies of the visual changes which occur in schizophrenia. They don't see the importance of changes in perception. Perhaps, too, their preoccupation with patients' life histories leaves them little time for these studies.

One schizophrenic tried to get admitted to a psychiatric ward because he thought others were talking about him, yet knew this was not so. At the same time he had visual disturbances and he decided he must be getting sick again. He was refused admittance, however, and told to go home "because you are normal."

There are two excellent ways for psychiatrists to become conscious of perceptual changes in patients. The first is long and arduous. It involves many years of experience with psychiatric patients, during which each is carefully examined for these changes. The second method, a faster and more effective one, is to take one of the hallucinogenic drugs such as LSD-25, mescalin or psilocybin, and study these changes at first hand. We think most psychiatrists would profit from the experience, and their understanding of their patients would improve.

Auditory hallucinations occur after schizophrenia is well established. The changes appear to occur in order as follows:

a. Patients become aware of their own thoughts.
b. They hear them in their head.
c. They hear them as if outside their head.
d. They hear voices.

The hallucinations can be anything from voices giving orders and conversations with God, to music, unearthly sounds and buzzing noises. There is no way of predicting in advance what the patient will hear. This will probably depend upon his personality, the part of the brain that is affected by the body chemical producing these changes, and other factors. The voices may belong to people known to the patient, alive or dead. They may teach the subject, or hold conversations with him. They may make fun of him or give him orders such as, "Do not eat any more." Religious communications have been very common, but in recent years sexual comments seem to have become more frequent.

The nature of the communication is not as important as the ability of the patient to act, or refrain from acting, on the advice given him. The only exception is the case of the patient who came to hospital in response to a voice which told her to.

A person may have the most vivid hallucinations, yet appear normal as long as he can refrain from doing what the voices tell him to, and telling others about them. One patient, a physically and mentally rugged individual, heard voices telling him as he shaved every morning, "Cut your throat, cut your throat." But he *knew* this was nonsense and carried on as if these voices did not exist.

This man had lost both legs in action in 1917 during the First World War and had made a splendid adjustment to this disaster. His schizophrenia did not develop until 1947, thirty years later.

One of the stages in treatment, therefore, is to convince patients not to tell others about their hallucinations.

3. CHANGES IN SENSES OF SMELL

Patients may become either more or less sensitive to odors. Since smell is an important factor in taste, any change in the former may lead to a change in the latter. The patient may become acutely aware of odors he normally did not notice before. Body odors may become exaggerated and unpleasant. Other people may smell strange. Consequently, patients may wash themselves excessively or insist that others do so.

Of course, hallucinations of the sense of smell can occur and in this case, patients will be aware of odors which are really not present. These hallucinations seem rare in schizophrenia but as questions about smell are not commonly asked, we really do not know. Patients will complain about them only when the changes are pronounced.

4. CHANGES IN SENSE OF TOUCH

These changes seem to occur less frequently than in any of the senses described above. Patients may become more or less sensitive to touch. Usually they become less sensitive to pain. Decrease in touch sensitivity is generally not troublesome unless the patient's job depends upon a keenness of touch.

But an increased sensitivity can be very troublesome. The feel of a fabric can be exaggerated until it feels like animal fur. There might be bizarre sensations, like the feeling that worms are crawling under one's skin. Unusual touch sensations may be interpreted as having electricity applied to one's person, being stuck with needles and so on.

There may be increased or decreased sensitivity in the genital organs, resulting in sexual delusions.

Normal subjects commonly experience the feeling of being out of the body when they take LSD-25. This usually occurs when the subject is so relaxed he is unaware of his own body. The medical explanation for this may be that messages from the outside of the body to the brain are temporarily suspended, and the patient's "perceived body" is distorted.

"Perceived body" is awareness of the limits of one's own body. This is undeveloped in babies, but well defined in adults. It is unlikely schizophrenic children have defective perceived body images and so easily run into solid objects. Also, if the body image is diffuse, patients can invade other people's "personal" space.

In their research in Weyburn Hospital, Dr. Osmond and Dr. R. Sommer, research psychologists, found that there is a space surrounding each person which, if invaded by another, makes him very anxious. You have seen some people talking face to face, while others are at least a yard away. The extent of personal space around each individual is determined psychologically and by the customs of the society in which he lives.

If a young female schizophrenic loses the ability to judge body image, she may unwittingly get too close to men and so appear to them to be forward or seductive, with many undesirable results. Staring at another is a violation of personal space and makes one feel anxious. One may feel threatened or "dominated" if an individual we dislike gets too close to us in conversation.

Sometimes, in another disturbance of "perceived body," the subject who has taken LSD-25 sees his own body from the outside as though he were on the ceiling looking down on himself, but this is rare. This also occurs with some schizophrenic patients. One patient was placed in a jail cell because of his asocial behavior. During this incarceration he woke up one day and, hearing footsteps in the corridor, went to his cell door to look out. In the corridor he saw himself pacing restlessly up and down. He examined himself, said, "I must be crazy," and retired to his cot to finish his nap.

5. TASTE CHANGES

In schizophrenia the proper balance of flavors is altered. Patients may become less sensitive to taste so that foods taste unusual. New tastes may occur.

The only dangerous changes are those which lead the patient to believe someone has tampered with the food. In our culture bitter things are often associated with medicines or poisons, and it is very likely that the common delusion of schizophrenics that they are being poisoned stems from the hallucinations that the food tastes bitter.

Dr. John Conolly in 1849 believed that many of his patients' delusions arose from disorders in taste perception. He reported many patients would not eat because foods had a coppery taste.

6. TIME CHANGES

We will include time as one of the important senses even though there seems to be no definite organ which deals with it. It is likely time perception is a function of the entire brain which acts as a computer integrating all sources of information from the senses to estimate the passing of time, for example, the eye sees day and night, sun, stars and shadow. The ear hears different noises at different times of the day, while the body feels hunger and other sensations from bladder, bowel, fatigued muscles and heartbeats. All these impulses, taken together, help us to tell whether it is morning, noon or night.

This skill has to be learned, and time- or clock-conscious societies force their members to learn it more thoroughly than others, although no human is ever free of the need to know that time is passing.

Few people realize how important the sense of time passing is to them until they are deprived of external aids such as wristwatches, or unless they find themselves in a world where time has lost its normal qualities, such as in the world of LSD-25. Today, when so many new demands are being made on our ability to perceive the passing of time, we can imagine the havoc which would result in our daily lives if we suddenly found ourselves unable to judge, or be aware of, time passing normally. Yet schizophrenics are continually living with a distorted time sense.

Patients in mental hospitals are frequently disoriented for time, possibly due to the lack of external aids which other people depend upon. The sense of days and weeks passing is normally diminished when one is removed from one's daily occupation. People on vacation and patients in hospital are more disoriented than they are at home. In general, calendars, daily newspapers and daily visitors help maintain orientation. But mental hospitals are not so well blessed.

One of our chronic schizophrenic patients was completely disoriented for time until the nurses were instructed to show her the calendar and daily newspaper and to ask her frequently the day of the week and the date. With these aids she soon became normally oriented.

In schizophrenia there can be very few changes in the sense of time passing, but their effects are very profound. In our research we have found that schizophrenics are more confused and muddled about time than any other patients except those cn confusional states, for example, in senility or toxic states of other illnesses. They seem to be in long slow delirium, resembling the state normals find themselves in when they take LSD-25.

Time may appear to pass very slowly, as in the hour spent listening to a dull lecture. Time may pass very quickly, as in the three hours spent in an interesting chess game or in hours of love which fly by in minutes. Time may stop altogether when there is no sensation of time passing at all.

Some catatonic patients seem to be suspended in time. When they recover from their catatonia (the state suffered by some schizophrenics when they do not move or speak) they can remember things that happened around them, but not the order in which they happened. Time is normally sequential. That is, "today" follows "yesterday" and is behind "tomorrow." It would be very disturbing if this normal flow of time were reversed. This happened to one of our subjects who, when given LSD, found himself drinking his coffee before the cup was lifted to his lips! We have not yet seen this in patients but we have not made a particular point of inquiring about it. We do not doubt it does occur, but it is rare. The order of events in schizophrenia, however, can be confused.

The changes may be of short or long duration and one may follow the other. A patient may sit down for a few moments, stay there several hours and "come to" thinking only moments have passed. Schizophrenics alternate between periods of time passing slowly, and time passing quickly. When it is passing slowly, they may be depressed. When it is passing quickly, they may be excited and elated. It is usually believed the mood sets the time sense, but there is no reason why the time sense cannot set the mood.

In fact, in hypnotic experiments which we will describe later, the mood was exactly correlated with the change in time passing. The slowing down of time movement produced depressed emotions. The speeding up of time produced euphoria, cheerfulness and even mania. When time was stopped, catatonia was produced.

It is surprising that so little attention has been paid to time perception in schizophrenia and its relationship to mood, even though this has long been a matter of general knowledge. It is also surprising that so little use has been made of this knowledge to develop diagnostic tests for schizophrenia.

ADDITIONAL NOTES ON PERCEPTUAL CHANGES

It is impossible to describe all the changes which can occur in the whole range of perceptions, nor would it be desirable to do so. For one's attention should not be directed to the details of the changes, but rather to the fact that the changes are present.

For anyone to function normally, each sense has to be linked smoothly and easily to all the others. We make judgments on the basis of what our senses tell us. If anything goes wrong with any one of our senses, our lives at home, at work and in the community can be seriously disrupted.

Some people experience a phenomenon called "synesthesia" which may be normal for them, but surprising and frightening for others. In synesthesia some people see a flash of light at the same time they hear a musical note.

This commonly happens when one has taken LSD-25 or its related compound, mescalin. It also occurs in schizophrenia. One may feel a pain in the chest at the same time one sees a flash of light. This can be very disturbing to patients and can easily lead them to believe they are being controlled by magic, or by the influence of others. One patient kept getting messages from the planets. Some patients have a feeling of omnipotence and power.

The first responsibility, when changes do occur, is to diagnose the presence of schizophrenia. In order to do this accurately, the simple fact that perceptual changes are absent or present is most important, and when they are present, a diligent inquiry must be made before schizophrenia is ruled out.

It is important to know the kind of perceptual changes which are present in order to treat the subject intelligently. Very often a proper explanation to the patient will weaken the emotional effects of the perceptual change and make life simpler for him.

Thought

We will not attempt to list all the varieties of change in thought which occur in schizophrenia. They may all be classified into two main categories: change in thought process and change in thought content.

1. CHANGES IN THOUGHT PROCESS

By process of thinking we refer to the act of putting thoughts into words in a logical manner. Ideas follow one another simply and logically, and are appropriate to the time and situation. Random and stray thoughts do occur, but they are under control and do not interfere with the normal flow of thinking. Memory for recent and remote events is adequate and the timing of one's thoughts are in tune with, and appropriate to, the group engaged in the conversation.

Any major change in brain function may disturb or disrupt this normal flow of thinking. The following changes in thinking have been found in schizophrenia:

(i) *There are no ideas whatever: the mind is blank.* This happens momentarily now and then to all of us. Repeated momentary blocks of this kind are called blocking. But when there are minutes or hours of blankness, it is highly pathological. One patient was mute. After many hours of trying to get him to talk, he blurted out that he could not talk, for his mind was blank. When he was given a book to read, he was able to read it aloud perfectly correctly. The words on the page were properly registered on his brain and properly reproduced as words, but he had no thoughts of his own to put into words.

(ii) *The process of thinking may be slowed down.* This is found more frequently in patients who are severely depressed, whether or not schizophrenia is present, and may be related to a slowing down of the sense of time passing. One schizophrenic patient spoke extremely slowly, and answered questions only after prolonged pauses. When her sense of time passing was speeded up by hypnotic suggestion, she was able to respond much more quickly and speak more rapidly for several weeks.

The opposite of this, a marked acceleration of thought and speech, is also found in schizophrenia although it is more typical of manic states. This may account for the increased brilliance of many young schizophrenic patients when their schizophrenia is just beginning.

(iii) *Thought processes may be so disturbed that one thought is followed by another which has no direct connection with it.* Thoughts may jump about at random. Bizarre thoughts may intrude and interfere with normal thought.

(iv) *Memory and recall may become so disturbed that clear thinking becomes impossible.*

Patients have described some of these changes to Dr. Andrew McGhie and Dr. James Chapman as follows:

Sometimes I can't concentrate because my brain is going too fast and at other times it is either going too slow or has stopped altogether. I don't mean that my mind becomes a blank, it just gets stuck in a rut when I am thinking over and over again about one thing. It's just as if there was a crack in the record.

I may be thinking quite clearly and telling someone something and suddenly I get stuck. What happens is that I suddenly stick on a word or an idea in my head and I just can't move past it. It seems to fill my mind and there's no room for anything else. This might go on for a while and suddenly it's over. Afterwards I get a feeling that I have been thinking very deeply about whatever it was, but often I can't remember what it was that has filled my mind so completely.

My trouble is that I've got too many thoughts. You might think about something, let's say that ashtray and just think, oh! yes, that's for putting my cigarette in, but I would think of it and then I would think of a dozen different things connected with it at the same time.

My mind's away. I have lost control. There are too many things coming into my head at once and I can't sort them out.

These are some of the changes that can occur in thought process. They are frequently found in schizophrenia. They are invariably present in well-established cases but they may not be present very early in the illness.

Because the patient cannot control idea or thoughts, or perceive normally, his speech is disturbed, leading some professionals to believe there is a "schizophrenic language." There are some writers in the psychiatric literature who even give the impression that they know and can even hold conversations in a schizophrenic language. This is another myth.

Dr. Osmond and Dr. Sommer tested patients in the Weyburn Mental Hospital, Saskatchewan, with the Word Association Test which was originally used by Sir Francis Galton in 1879. The test is completely objective and can be given and scored by an untrained technician.

Dr. Osmond and Dr. Sommer became interested in this question while studying autobiographies of mental patients. When they compared these to books by former prisoners, they found that they could hardly read some prison books without a glossary because of the special language of prisoners. But there was no special language among mental patients. They felt this could explain the lack of organized social activity among schizophrenics, and the fact that schizophrenic patients did not organize mutinies, riots or protests.

In their studies with patients they found that schizophrenics not only had less in common in word associations than nonschizophrenic patients and normals, but that they did not understand one another's speech better than anyone else did. In fact, they found that patients were intolerant of the delusional and incoherent speech of other patients, and only paid attention when their fellow patients talked more or less normally. Patients sometimes complained about "crazy talk" by other patients and even walked out of meetings and group thdrapy sessions if there was too much of it.

They found that though the speech of schizophrenics may appear bizarre to us, they were actually responding to information received through their senses. Thus, rather than having a language of their own, they associate with their own associations to the words given them. Furthermore, as additional proof, a schizophrenic's associations to the same word may vary.

This leads us to believe there is no schizophrenic language, but that the schizophrenic's disjointed, rambling and often incoherent speech is another symptom of the schizophrenic process which has broken every line of contact with the world.

These are some of the changes that can occur in thought process. They are very frequently found in schizophrenia. They are invariably present in well-established cases, but they may not be present early in the illness.

2. CHANGES IN THOUGHT CONTENT

Everyone has wrong ideas. Superstitions, beliefs in certain "miracle" foods, prejudices against groups, extraordinary belief in one's own abilities are examples of commonly held wrong ideas.

We may go along quite contentedly with these ideas for most of our lives, particularly if most people in our society share them with us. When our wrong ideas conform to ideas generally accepted in the community, we are not sick even though other societies believe they are abnormal. For example, enormous numbers of men believe in racial superiority, while enormous numbers of other men believe this is a delusion. Yet the individuals who share this widely held belief are normal in their own society.

But at some time or another we may have to ask ourselves, is this idea true? Does it make sense? Is it normal to think that way?

We can decide for ourselves whether our ideas are true or normal by testing them. We can search for supporting evidence. We can compare them with the consensus of ideas in the community. We may then find our ideas are indeed wrong or different, but that we cannot help believing them. In that case we have to decide whether we want to keep our ideas even though they are wrong, or whether we want to change them.

If our ideas interfere with our jobs, with our relationships with relatives and friends and with our general effectiveness in our community, then we must examine them closely and decide either to take the consequences or to reject the ideas.

Many schizophrenics at one time or another in the course of their illness also have wrong ideas, but these are more extreme and may fluctuate. They may believe that someone has poisoned them or that they are victims of some community plot. This of course is not so, yet they may develop a long line of logical reasoning to explain why they believe this is so.

When he is well, the schizophrenic is able to judge whether his observations are true or not. But when he is sick his judgment is impaired. This, together with the changes in perception which characterize his illness, can lead to an infinite number of bizarre and unusual changes in thought. Again we must remind the reader that thought can be considered abnormal only if it differs markedly from the culture one is in.

We do not mean the kind of culture which refers to art or literature, nor do we mean a "cultured" person who is well versed in these matters. By culture we mean the total number of factors which have moulded or shaped the person in which he has grown and lived. Westerners grow up in a western culture of competition and judging status and prestige by wealth and accomplishment. North American Indians had varying cultures, where status meant different things in different tribes. Thus, a paranoid whose thoughts may be bizarre in our culture, is normal in a community where everyone else's ideas are also more or less paranoid.

It is relatively unimportant to know all the kinds of content changes which can occur in schizophrenia. There is hardly any idea which cannot be imagined and undoubtedly these have been found among schizophrenics. But if the ideas become extreme and unusually different from the thinking of people around them, they may be a symptom of schizophrenia.

Mood

Again few changes are possible, but these may vary. One may be depressed, normal in mood, too happy or completely lacking in feeling, that is flat or uninterested. The mood may not be consistent with the thought content expressed by the subject in his speech, and in this case may seem inappropriate to the observer.

Depression is the most common change in mood.

Everyone at times is depressed, expecially when one is sick, or frustrated, or has failed in some endeavor. In fact, it is so common that most people are convinced every depression must be the result of some failure, some reverse or some clear physical disease like infectious hepatitis (jaundice).

It is very difficult to convince many patients that the depression is primary and may occur in the absence of a precipitating event. Nearly all patients and most psychiatrists search ceaselessly for a reason and this search, which is so often fruitless and degrading, is aided and abetted by careless professional probing.

Depression is often the earliest symptom of schizophrenia, just as it is the first symptom of many other illnesses. Whenever depression occurs in a young person where there is no physical illness or other clear reason for it, schizophrenia should be suspected.

The depression (sadness) may come on slowly, endure for several days or weeks, and then vanish until the next episode. The subjects are then hounded by inexplicable moods of despair and irritability. When this occurs together with clear perceptual changes, the diagnosis can be made early.

But when depression occurs alone as the first symptom, the patient is not so fortunate. It is likely he will then be diagnosed as a depression or an anxiety neurosis for many years. The unfortunate schizophrenic will then fall into the group of depressions who within ten years are clearly schizophrenic, or in the group who respond to ECT (electric shock treatment) or to anti-depressant drugs with a gratifying change of mood but, to the horror of their doctor, now appear schizophrenic.

Meanwhile, many valuable years have been lost during which the patient could have been given specific treatment and spared useless therapies.

The period of depression may be followed by a feeling of

euphoria, when the patient feels much too happy when all circumstances are taken into account. But these periods of elation are few. The usual story is to have periods of depression followed by periods of normality. If the moods are too short and follow each other rapidly, especially in young people, schizophrenia is very likely the reason.

Over the past ten years psychiatry has given more emphasis to mood swings while continuing to ignore perceptual changes and thought disorder. If mood swings are present they are invariably diagnosed bipolar or manic depressive psychosis. Perceptual changes are minimized by ascribing them to a type of delirium induced by the manic state and thought disorder is now considered a symptom characteristic of this affective disease. This belief is reinforced by the fact that a few patients do show features of both diseases and that their moods are stabilized by lithium. Many equate recovery by lithium as the definitive diagnosis of manic depressive psychosis.

During the early stages of the illness the depression is always appropriate to the patient's circumstances. This, too, makes diagnosis difficult since many psychiatrists wait for the depression to become inappropriate before they will entertain the diagnosis of schizophrenia. But this delay is very dangerous, for the disease becomes well entrenched and chronic before the mood becomes inappropriate enough to satisfy the psychiatrist. No research has come to our attention which shows how long it takes for a schizophrenic's depression to become inappropriate, but it must be several years.

The most common inappropriateness is flatness, in which the patient feels neither depression nor happiness. He feels no emotion at all and is completely apathetic. This can be a disturbing symptom for subjects who once did feel appropriately, but if it occurs very early in life, and has been present many years, they get used to it and eventually find it quite tolerable. It is probably easier to endure than the severe tension and depression which usually precedes it.

Upon recovering, however, the ability to feel emotion often returns, and this too can be disturbing to patients. Dr. Hoffer and Dr. Osmond have often seen this happen in patients who were receiving adequate treatment with nicotinic acid. It is a mistake in this case to assume that the occurrence of anxiety and tension indicates the disease has recurred.It is on the contrary a heartening sign. The patient's tension can be easily controlled with anti-tension compounds, which can be slowly withdrawn usually after a month or so.

The flatness of moods is puzzling. It is very characteristic of schizophrenia but there is no adequate explanations for it. It is possible it is responsible for the inappropriateness of mood for, if a person can feel no mood, in time he will lose the ability to judge what his mood should be. Many schizophrenics compensate intellectually for the inability to feel emotions by observing others in a social and group situation, and role-playing the appropriate mood. If the others are sad or gay, they feel they must also be sad or gay and act accordingly. This is very hard on them and may lead them to avoid group situations.

One beneficial effect of this flatness of mood is that it probably keeps many schizophrenics from killing themselves. It is well known that many severely depressed people do kill themselves but it not generally known that schizophrenics also have a very high suicide rate and it might even be higher if they did not have some flatness of mood.

Research in Saskatchewan and elsewhere shows that out of any group of schizophrenics, about 0.2 per cent will kill themselves each year. If one started with one thousand fresh cases of schizophrenia, one would expect that two will die each year from suicide, whether they have or have not received psychiatric treatment. The only exception we know of is the treatment program which includes nicotinic acid. Out of over three hundred schizophrenic patients treated adequately with nicotinic acid, who have been followed up in Saskatchewan for nearly ten years, there have been no suicides.

With the flatness of mood, therefore, it appears as if the disease itself acts as a poor tranquilizer. This will be discussed in a subsequent chapter. The only hallucinogens (drugs capable of producing hallucinations as in schizophrenia) which reproduce this peculiar mood flatness are adrenochrome and adrenaline which are probably present in the body, and which we think are somehow responsible for the disease process called schizophrenia. This hypothesis will also be discussed in the next chapter.

Activity

It should not be surprising that changes in perception, thought and mood should lead to changes in behavior. We will not describe these for they lead directly from the other changes. If a person feels he is being spied upon, it seems only natural he should take some action, either defensive or offensive.

We wish only to discuss briefly the common belief that schizophrenics are dangerous. They are, indeed, somewhat more dangerous to themselves than they would be if they were not schizophrenic, but they are not more dangerous to other people.

The risk of homicide among schizophrenics is no greater than it is for non-schizophrenics. Nevertheless, this belief is so well engrained it has until recently been an article of faith for mental hospital architects, society and even for nursing staff. This is one reason mental hospitals have been built like fortresses and jails. The best evidence that this is false is the fact that one or two rather small female nurses can herd as many as forty to sixty or more chronic schizophrenics.

There are, of course, isolated incidents of homicide. These result from certain delusions, especially when the hospital staff do not treat the patient appropriately. It is a general rule that a violent aggressive patient is a sign of poor psychiatric treatment. Most modern mental hospitals have done away with physical restraints, cuffs, guards, etc., with great success.

The behavior of schizophrenic patients is predictable when one takes the trouble to find out, not only what they think, but what they perceive.

Self-Diagnosis

These are the highlights of the changes which occur in schizophrenia. No one patient has them all nor do they remain the same from month to month. We do not advise subjects to diagnose themselves, but we do advise them to familiarize themselves with the symptoms and, if they in any way have similar ones, to seek help. This is the subject's responsibility, just as much as it is the responsibility of a woman to be aware of lumps in her breast, which could be cancerous, or of anyone to know that excess consumption of liquids, too much urine, loss of weight and weakness could indicate *diabetes mellitus*.

A second way of diagnosing oneself is to become familiar with self-accounts written by schizophrenic patients who have recovered. For this purpose a bibliography is included at the end of this book.

A third way is to complete the HOD test* (Hoffer-Osmond Diagnostic test). Any person who scores very high on this test should decide, not that he is schizophrenic, but that, if he has symptoms which lead him to believe he is ill, he should be examined by a psychiatrist.

A normal person who has no symptoms will not score highly. Young people under sixteen tend to score much higher than older people and should not be given the test. The test and its interpretation should be left to a psychiatrist.

There will be some who maintain that no one should even be allowed to suspect that he or she might have schizophrenia. This is incompatible with modern scientific principles. There should be no secrecy in medicine. The days of guilds, Latin prescriptions and other secret devices are long past. In fact, in our experience, patients do appreciate having their suspicions about themselves either denied or confirmed. We have had several patients who were quite certain they were schizophrenic, and they were correct. They were easily treated with nicotinic acid alone. It is very rare for patients to be disturbed when given the diagnosis if the psychiatrist himself is not frightened. But the diagnosis must be followed by a description of schizophrenia as an illness which will respond to treatment as the main component of it is chemical.

Alcoholics Anonymous has discovered it is good for alcoholics to hear from other alcoholics about their problems. AA literature also follows this principle. Thus *The Grapevine*, the official monthly publication of AA, contains many interesting accounts written by alcoholics who have recovered.

These serve two purposes: (1) they provide security by consensus: that is, patients realize there are many others with similar problems; (2) they are given examples of people equally sick who have recovered. It is quite likely a similar compilation of case

*This is a simple card sort test which helps to differentiate schizophrenia patients from others. It is so designed that high scores indicate schizophrenia is present.

histories would be equally useful for schizophrenic patients who would be encouraged to read them.

Another more sophisticated test is the Experiential World Inventory developed by Dr. Moneim El-Meligi and one of us (H.O.) available from Robert Mullaly, Ph.D., Intuition Press, P.O. Box 404, Keene, NH 03431. It follows the principles described here and used by the HOD test, but it is a more sensitive diagnostic instrument and is very helpful when the HOD results are equivocal. It will probably be the psychologist's diagnostic test, while the HOD will remain the psychiatrist's office test.

CHAPTER III

CAUSES OF SCHIZOPHRENIA

T HERE are few things in life which have one cause. There are
no diseases where single causes operate. On the contrary, there is
no limit to the number and diversity of causes which may work
together in producing any disease.

A simple example will show how complicated this matter can
be. Suppose a man walks hurriedly from his house to catch his
bus to work, after having had a fight with his wife. He stumbles
over his son's bicycle lying on the sidewalk and fractures a leg.

What was the cause of the leg fracture? Here is a list of events
which might be considered causal, to illustrate how various
interested theorists might look at it:

The organicist—the fracture came from the act of falling.

The biochemist—the bone may have been weak due to loss of
calcium, for example, when lacking Vitamin D.

The personality theorist—the fracture resulted because the
man had a personality which prevented him from having a
mature relationship with his wife. As a result, his argument with
her so enraged him that he blindly strode from the house and fell,
breaking a leg.

The sociologist—the man's need to arrive at work on time
created a situation where there was insufficient time for the man
to complete his argument with his wife, i.e., the socio-economic
situation resulted in the leg fracture.

The psychoanalyst—the husband had not freed himself from a
dependent relationship with his mother. This unresolved
situation was transferred to his wife to whom he related as a
mother figure. The argument with his wife reawakened anxiety
induced by the trauma of birth ("his first separation from a

dependent situation") which was reawakened by fears of separation since. The argument with his wife brought out his latent hostility and his need for a dependency relationship.

Therefore, he subconsciously denied the existence of his son's bicycle, thus proving to himself he was not really an adult after all. The fall and fracture were thus mechanisms for gaining, once more, the security of the womb. The fracture was a small price to pay. This hypothesis seems stronger when it is realized that the husband, when he fell down, also momentarily achieved a fetal situation.

The demonologist—the demon had taken possession of the man who had bargained his soul for profit. But this produced great conflict before the profits began to accrue. The devil caused him to trip and fall to remind him of his pledge.

It is quite clear that in this simple situation anyone looking at it can come up with a satisfactory cause. Some might see the fracture as the work of the devil, others as an act of punishment. It is, therefore, not logical to talk about causes until one understands clearly exactly what relevance these causes have to the problem which is presented.

Well, then, what is the problem? The answer is simple. The problem is to treat the condition. Physicians are interested primarily in curing patients if possible. They are interested in causes only if this leads to better treatment. In the example cited, none of the causes are relevant with one possible exception, and that is, if the fracture was really due to a pre-existing and alterable weakness of the bone. But in any event the first thing the physician does is to ease the pain, prevent excessive loss of blood, reduce the possibility of infection and set the broken bone. That is, the condition is treated—no more and no less.

We can, therefore, divide causes into two main groups: (*a*) those that are most readily treated (these we will call the most modifiable causes; (*b*) those that are merely contributing factors.

In the example above, the most modifiable cause, the one most easily treated, is the fracture. This must be set. Usually that will be sufficient. But if the man broke his leg repeatedly other factors will have to be investigated.

We will divide the causes or factors which lead to schizophrenia in the same way. We consider that the most easily treated factors are biochemical due to genetic influences, and that secondary or contributing factors are all those which may be considered psychological, sociological and psycho-physiological.

Before anyone can get schizophrenia, his body "factory," which uses up chemicals and produces other chemicals, must be different from that of a normal subject in that it must have the capacity to go out of order for some reason, and start biochemical changes in motion. This is an essential cause of schizophrenia. Without it, the disease cannot occur. With it, it may occur, but it also may not, just as everyone susceptible to tuberculosis does not develop tuberculosis.

Once the process is established, the patient has schizophrenia. How he acts, what he thinks, will be decided by the secondary or contributing factors—the kind of perceptual changes which occur, the culture in which he lives and his own personality. It is important to know what these are if one is to treat the patient adequately, for they mould the disease process and determine the content of the illness. But there is very little evidence to support the claim that they can trigger the disease.

Biochemical Hypotheses

All emotions have biochemical as well as psychological elements. A biochemical theory of schizophrenia, therefore, must account for the disease in the following way:

1. The biochemical mechanism involved in the theory should be related in a logical way to the biochemical factors which we know have something to do with anxiety or stress. There should be a clear relationship between the chemicals and the emotions even if the latter are only contributing factors to the disease.

2. There must be a biochemical upset in patients and none in normal subjects.

3. The substances which come from the abnormal chemical operations must themselves be able to produce changes in normal subjects similar to those found in schizophrenia.

4. The presence of the biochemical changes should account for the clinical peculiarities of schizophrenia. They must produce the resistance to histamine, freedom from allergies and marked resistance to medical shock that schizophrenics enjoy.

5. The product of these biochemical abnormalities should produce changes in the brain which can account for perceptual,

thought and mood changes which are found in schizophrenia.

6. Restoring biochemical normality should help cure the patient.

Various theories have been proposed to explain schizophrenia on a biochemical basis, and of these, two have emerged as the main ones. The first, the adrenochrome-adrenolutin theory developed in Saskatchewan, is the only one which satisfies all of the above requirements. Professor R. Heath's taraxein hypothesis satisfies most of them.

The adrenochrome-adrenolutin theory was first developed publicly in 1952 and is based on, or originates from, the amino-acid called tyrosine. This is a simple amino-acid from which skin pigment and the hormones, noradrenaline and adrenaline, as well as other constituents, are made.

Professor Heath's taraxein hypothesis comes from this theory, and may eventually be found to be related to it, although no connection has been found as yet. The two theories may be complementary, each accounting for a portion of the biochemical pathology. It is clear they are not antagonistic. All toxic theories may be said to be variants of the taraxein theory, but Professor Heath was the first to extract taraxein, inject it into animals, including man, give it a name and begin to study its structure. He must, therefore, be given priority in this matter.

Another biochemical hypothesis is called the serotonin hypothesis. Serotonin comes from another amino-acid called tryptophane. It does not meet any of the above standards, but it has received serious consideration. It seems to be running into a decline, if a decrease in the number of papers published on it recently can be considered an indication. Other suggestions have been made that other products of tryptophane are somehow involved, but they have not yet been examined adequately.

We do not consider that any of the theories presented here are perfect. The future will probably see the development of more satisfactory theories, and the ones presented here may then seem simple and naïve. But hindsight always allows one to consider what has gone before as naïve. We hope the theories we discuss in this book will some day be markedly altered and new and better ones introduced, for this is the way of science. Biochemists continually challenge each other for change, in sharp contrast to the psychoanalyst whose greatest terror is that Freud might be proven wrong.

Adrenochrome-Adrenolutin Hypothesis

Body hormones are constantly changing into other hormones. Each new hormone has its own structure and role in the building of the final structure of the body, and helping it function. Body hormones are carried by the blood to all parts of the body, on which they have a direct effect. Some affect growth. Some affect digestion. Some affect moods. They may be necessary to the normal function of a tissue. Chemicals may join forces with other chemicals to produce still other effects.

As long as they go about their business in a routine fashion, the individual remains well. But when, for some reason they change routine, or the normal balance of chemicals is changed, the person becomes ill.

The adrenochrome-adrenolutin theory is based on the assumption that certain chemicals stop following the normal procedures, and the result is schizophrenia. It involves the study of products of the adrenal gland, a little triangular-shaped organ weighing only one ounce, which sits on top of each kidney.

The adrenal gland is made up of an inner part called the medulla, and outer part called the cortex. In the central area, the medulla, a hormone called noradrenaline is made, and from this comes adrenaline, a hormone important to the emotions. Adrenaline flows from the inner area through the cortex into the bloodstream.

Scattered through the body are tissues similar to the adrenal medulla which can also make adrenaline. When the adrenal medulla is destroyed or removed, these tissues begin to grow and soon put out nearly the original supply, so that the body is never without it.

In an emergency situation, adrenaline acts as a co-ordinator of the many mechanisms required for use. It helps to mobilize the biological resources for fight or flight.

When a man is attacked by a bear or by a sabre-tooth tiger, for example, he is immediately ready for action, whether or not he is afraid. A few seconds later adrenaline and other hormones are pouring into the bloodstream and the body is soon flooded with them. It seems likely there is a fine balance of psychological and biochemical factors as the following changes occur.

The rate of breathing is increased. The heart rate goes up and the pulse count is faster. Blood pressure goes up. Sugar is poured into the blood. Blood is channeled from the internal organs which are not essential for the defence operations—bowel, stomach, etc.—to the aid of the muscles needed for the hard work ahead. Pain sensitivity is reduced. The blood is ready to stop bleeding more quickly, if it occurs.

There are many other changes, and the person is now ready for fight or flight. A sustained effort is needed, though, and here slower mechanisms come into play. The final result is to increase the chances of survival.

Once the drama is over, the individual is psychologically relieved or relaxed, the hormone production slows down, and the body gets rid of the extra supply of used chemicals either by destroying them or excreting them.

Adrenaline also plays a role in the emotions in smaller quantities. There is good evidence that it helps the person feel anxious and may play a role in depression.

This hormone turns into a very toxic and changeable hormone called adrenochrome. Adrenochrome can be seen as part of the red pigment coloring adrenaline when this substance is allowed to stand in water solution in the open air. It has been, and is, easily made in the laboratory as a dark crystalline material. In its pure form it manifests itself as beautiful, sharp, needle-like crystals which have a brilliant sheen. When the crystals are powdered, it appears as a bright red powder, which dissolves quickly in water to form a blood-red solution. It is very reactive, and combines quickly with many other chemicals. There is substantial evidence, both direct and indirect, that adrenochrome is also formed in the body. More work is required to prove this to everyone's satisfaction.

Adrenochrome in the test tube and in the body can, in turn, be changed into two new compounds. One of these is harmless, and is called 5,6 dihydroxy-N-methyl-indole (hereafter referred to as dihydroxyindole or leuco-adrenochrome) and the other is poisonous and is called adrenolutin.

Adrenolutin is a bright yellow crystalline material with an orange tinge when pure. Impure preparations develop a greenish color. The darker the material, the more impure it is. It is difficult to dissolve in water. When an ultra-violet lamp shines on it, it glows with a beautiful blue-white color.

The other hormone in this triangle, dihydroxyindole, consists of small flattish crystals which are slightly off-white color. They dissolve easily in water to form a colorless solution.

Large amounts of dihydroxyindole have been given to animals

and men, and if any changes have occurred, they have been beneficial ones. It is possible this compound works against adrenaline to create a balance which keeps the person from becoming too tense or irritable. We have elsewhere suggested that tension or anxiety depends upon how much dihydroxyindole is present as compared with adrenaline. If there is too much adrenaline and too little dihydroxyindole, we suggest that the person will be too anxious.

This whole process, then, from adrenaline to adrenochrome to dihydroxyindole or adrenolutin is the essence of the adreno-chrome-adrenolutin theory of schizophrenia, and can be sketched as follows:

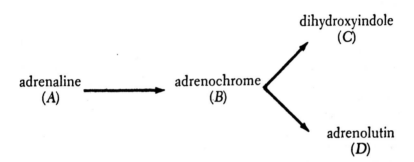

We suggested many years ago that the normal pathway of these changes is from A to B to C, and that if A and C are present in normally balanced quantities, the subject will be neither too tense or too relaxed. Adrenochrome (B) reacts very quickly and probably does not remain free in the body very long.

In schizophrenics, however, for reasons still unknown, the pathway is from A to B to D. Adrenolutin provides some relaxation, but it interferes with normal chemical reactions in the brain, and the process of schizophrenia is under way.

If this theory is correct, we can expect certain things to happen. In fact, it is important to test these ideas to see if these consequences do occur. And if they do, then belief in the adrenochrome hypothesis must be strengthened and the theory more widely accepted. The three main sets of consequences of this theory are:

1. If the theory as shown is true, then adrenochrome and adrenolutin, when injected into animals and man, will reproduce some of the essential features of schizophrenia.

2. If the theory as shown is true, then adrenochrome and adrenolutin or their products are present in the body. When a person has schizophrenia, they are present in greater concentrations.

3. If the theory as shown is true, then any mechanism which reduces the formation of adrenolutin or adrenochrome, or which removes them from the body altogether when they are formed, or counteracts their effects, will cure schizophrenia.

The evidence so far established supports all three suppositions. Much more evidence is needed, but there is enough now to make it impossible to prove otherwise. Following is the evidence that all these expected consequences of the adrenochrome theory do occur.

1. ADRENOCHROME AND ADRENOLUTIN PRODUCE CHANGES IN ANIMALS AND MAN

The first human studies with adrenochrome were started in 1952 in Saskatchewan. Usually new chemicals are first given to animals to test toxicity and determine their effects on the body. But no animals were then available and we were. The first studies were completed on ourselves.

One of our first clues to adrenochrome as a possible villain in the body came from a severe asthmatic. Before coming to Saskatchewan in 1951, Dr. Osmond and a young colleague at St. George's Hospital, London, England, Dr. John Smythies, had experimented with mescalin and noted that the experience resembled that of some schizophrenics. While listening to a recording of a mescalin experiment, this subject remarked that things like that sometimes happened to him. If he took very large amounts of adrenaline, as he sometimes did, the world changed; he had colored visions with his eyes shut, and feelings of unreality. In Regina, Dr. E. Asquith later told us that during the war, pinkish adrenaline was used during anaesthesia, and when the patients revived they had disturbances including hallucinations.

Early in 1952 we called upon Professor Duncan Hutcheon, Professor D. MacArthur and Dr. V. Woodford, of the University Medical School in Saskatoon, and asked for their help. We mentioned pinkish adrenaline and Professor Hutcheon suggested adrenochrome, which comes from adrenaline and resembles mescalin. Professor MacArthur showed that it could be related to every hallucinogen then known if one examined its chemical structure.

Professor Hutcheon made our first small supply of good adrenochrome and, before he left Saskatchewan in early 1953, we had a model of schizophrenia from these early experiments, starting with ourselves and our wives.

Dr. Hoffer was the first to take adrenochrome and Dr. Osmond the second. Ten minutes after taking it, Dr. Osmond noticed that the ceiling had changed color and that the lighting had become brighter. He closed his eyes and saw a brightly colored pattern of dots which gradually formed fish-like shapes. He felt he was at the bottom of the sea or in an aquarium with a shoal of brilliant fishes. At one moment he thought he was a sea anemone in this pool. He was amazed when he was given psychological tests and asked to relate what was happening. He was given a Van Gogh self-portrait to examine.

He later wrote, "I have never seen a picture so plastic and alive. Van Gogh gazed at me from the paper, crop-headed, with hurt, mad eyes and seemed to be three dimensional. I felt that I could stroke the cloth of his coat and that he might turn around in his frame."

When he left the laboratory he "found the corridors outside sinister and unfriendly. I wondered what the cracks in the floor meant and why there were so many of them. Once we got out-of-doors the hospital buildings, which I know well, seemed sharp and unfamiliar. As we drove through the streets the houses appeared to have some special meaning, but I couldn't tell what it was. In one window I saw a lamp burning and I was astonished by its grace and brilliance. I drew my friends' attention to it but they were unimpressed."

The second time Dr. Osmond took adrenochrome he had no feelings for human beings. "As we drove back to Abe's house a pedestrian walked across the road in front of us. I thought we might run him down, and watched with detached curiosity. I had no concern for the victim. We did not knock him down. I began to wonder whether I was a person any more and to think that I might be a plant or a stone. As my feeling for these inanimate objects increased, my feeling for and my interest in humans diminished. I felt indifferent towards humans and had to curb myself from making unpleasant personal remarks about them."

The next day he attended a scientific meeting, and during it he wrote this note: "Dear Abe, this damn stuff is still working. The odd thing is that stress brings it on, after about fifteen minutes. I have this 'glass wall, other side of the barrier' feeling. It is fluctuant, almost intangible, but I know it is there. It wasn't there three-quarters of an hour ago; the stress was the minor one of getting the car. I have a feeling that I don't know anyone here; absurd but unpleasant. Also some slight ideas of reference arising from my sensation of oddness. I have just begun to wonder if my hands are writing this, crazy of course."

Later he found he could not relate distance and time. "We had coffee at a wayside halt and here I became disturbed by the covert glances of a sinister looking man."

The two observers later wrote, "The change in H.O. marked by strong preoccupation with inanimate objects, by a marked refusal to communicate with us, and by strong resistance to our requests, was in striking contrast with H.O.'s normal social behavior."

Experiences like these, and like the one described by a young man, whom we call Mr. Kovish, led us to believe that we were on the right track. Mr. Kovish was in his middle thirties, friendly, intelligent and with a lively sense of humor. After subsequent interviews with him, we felt we had no reason to doubt his story.

Mr. Kovish occasionally suffered from asthma, for which he had taken adrenaline by inhalation regularly for at least ten years. One night in mid-1956 he found himself without adrenaline, many miles from home. He stopped at a drug store and the druggist said that all he had was one bottle but that it was quite discolored. He seemed hesitant to sell it but Mr. Kovish bought it anyway. While driving later that night he felt alert and wakeful, but had some difficulty in judgement and some bizarre thoughts. His vision was distorted. The road which was very familiar to him looked different. He felt alert to an extreme and pulled off the road. This seemed very strange to him.

This was the beginning of an experience which thoroughly frightened him. He suspected he was becoming mentally ill and he was ashamed of what was happening to him. He did not, however, associate these changes with the adrenaline, and continued to take it for about a month at various intervals until he had finished the bottle.

"I have always felt myself to be a normal individual—unneurotic and with a zest for living," he later wrote to the authors. "It was, therefore, quite a shock to me to find one day that I had suddenly become an individual who: (1) saw the world as through a distorted glass: I sought to interpret the visual distortions as being due to strange mental processes; (2) became quite anxious and depressive; (3) had compulsive thoughts; (4) began to doubt myself and my sanity . . . Had I known that I was going to have an artificially induced psychosis, I am sure the severity of the consequences would not have been felt because, not knowing the origin, I ascribed them to psychic difficulties, and this led me deeper into my feelings of unrest. I went into a tailspin, and perhaps this had something to do with the length of the effect. I also should mention that I was in a personally stressful situation which might have been a contributing factor."

Mr. Kovish described some of his symptoms as "tendency toward fixed thinking, feelings of excitement for no apparent reason, surroundings especially people (men much more so than women) looked peculiar, including pictures in newspapers."

He remembers being bothered by groups of people. "I felt that there was something distorted or different appearing about them. This was not localized to any one person. There was a strangeness about seeing groups of people which had a somewhat frightening effect on me. I noticed distortion in many things, some animate and some inanimate . . . I saw people more or less like I have seen before, except that they impressed me differently, and this was very frightening . . . I could find no logical reason for this strange thing that was happening to me and I spiralled downwards to the depth of despair at having lost my mind and I felt that that was a very disgraceful and shameful thing to do."

He was able to reconcile himself to familiar people very easily by telling himself, "Now look, you have seen these people before. They are not really changed. They haven't changed. It's got to be you."

He suffered anxiety, depression, compulsive thoughts which had no relation to reality. He had bizarre thoughts which seemed to be connected with the strangeness of the way people appeared to him. Internal excitement plagued him. He had never had any fear of flying through storm or any other stressful situation. Now he was extremely anxious in an airplane.

He was "too charged up" at times to sleep at nights, and

experienced "uncertain visual patterns and shapes a few times" before dropping off to sleep, which he hadn't experienced before or since. What was more, he had no asthma or wheezing at night under any circumstances, except once when he was at the home of a friend who had dogs; and was completely without asthmatic symptoms even after heavy exercises. "It can be summed up by saying I felt like one is supposed to feel when they have had a lot of adrenaline."

He was extremely irritable, felt low and could no longer participate in family life, such as playing with the children and talking things over with his wife. While discussing this with a friend one day he casually mentioned the adrenaline. She immediately reminded him of R. W. Gerard's article in *Science* on "Biological Roots of Psychiatry" in which he discussed breakdown products of adrenaline as causing temporary psychoses. In re-reading Gerard's article he found a description that seemed to fit his feelings exactly.

He wrote to the author of this article, who referred him to an article we had written. In this article he found more specific details which helped sustain him to the end of his distressing symptoms. When the experience was over his asthma was gone.

This story had exciting implications. Outside of a laboratory, unsuspecting and unprepared, a normal man had taken "bad" adrenaline and as a result had suffered all the classic symptoms of schizophrenia for several weeks. He had no advance knowledge of what the drug would do to him and was, in fact, reluctant to admit that it had been the cause of his troubles.

Those close to him, who had always seen him as a man with good reserves of humor and optimism even when things seemed difficult, were very surprised and disturbed when he seemed so unlike himself. They had never seen him like that before. His account furthermore resembled in many ways famous accounts of schizophrenic illness and experiments with drugs such as mescalin, LSD-25, adrenochrome, adrenolutin and others.

After hearing of the effect of inhaled discolored adrenaline on Mr. Kovish, we began exploratory experiments with inhaled adrenolutin. We were the first to take adrenolutin, but under the influence of the drug we had no insight into our own behavior. The third volunteer to take it, a normally friendly outgoing young man, alarmed his family with violent temper outbursts, delusions, suspiciousness and other behavior typical of schizophrenia.

Most of the subjects reacted to adrenochrome and adrenolutin. The most striking changes were changes in personality which continued up to two weeks in several volunteers. There was no insight, and even though the subjects were aware that they had taken these chemicals, and remembered having taken them, they assumed the changes in themselves had nothing to do with the drugs. Several subjects became temporarily psychotic and one had to be admitted to a mental hospital for several months of treatment.

We found that in human volunteers adrenochrome or adrenolutin produced the following changes:

Changes in perception: These are subtle, but no less serious, when small doses are used. With thirty mg. or more placed under the tongue, visual hallucinations are produced which may be as clear and destinct as those experienced with LSD. Furthermore, all the changes found in schizophrenics as described in chapter II may occur with adrenochrome.

Changes in thought: These are also similar to those found in schizophrenia.

Changes in mood: In most cases the subjects were depressed but sometimes they were too relaxed or flat.

Our conclusions, based upon these few original studies, have been confirmed by other research workers in the United States, Germany and Czechoslovakia. They might not, in themselves, be adequate, but they receive very strong support from the results of experiments with animals.

Adrenochrome and adrenolutin have been given to spiders, mice, rats, cats, dogs, rabbits and monkeys. These studies have been carried out in Sweden, Russia, Czechoslovakia, Germany, Switzerland, Canada and the United States. These compounds have shown activity in animals in every study except one, where adrenochrome was used in too small quantities. In every other study, animal behavior as a result of the injection of adrenochrome and adrenolutin, was altered markedly.

Russian experimenters, using sensitive methods, showed that very small amounts of the poisonous substances given to trained monkeys rendered them incapable of carrying out procedures they could easily perform before and after.

In Moscow, scientists trained monkeys to work for their food by handling an apparatus which released a banana if they did it right. They had to press a button, pull a cord and perform other tasks in order, and if they were done accurately, the banana which came out as a result was their reward.

When given one mg. of adrenochrome, they were no longer able to go through the routine, even if they were as hungry as before. But they knew what a banana was, and they knew they were hungry, and if a banana was placed beside their cage they reached out and picked it up. Thus they were able to perform at a very simple level, but had lost the ability to carry out more complicated tasks which they were able to do well before taking adrenochrome, and after they had recovered from it. The adrenochrome also made them bad-tempered, boorish and lacking in social graces.

Work at the University of Saskatchewan showed that rats given adrenochrome were not able to learn as readily as normal animals, and they forgot what they had learned more quickly. One could look upon them as rats that had become retarded because of adrenochrome. There are few who doubt that adrenochrome is active in animals or in man, and it is now included among the family of compounds known as hallucinogens—compounds like mescaline and LSD-25 capable of producing psychological changes in man.

2. ADRENOCHROME METABOLISM AND SCHIZOPHRENIA

Adrenochrome has not been isolated from living tissue, but there are indications that it soon will be. J. Axelrod, one of the scientists who previously maintained adrenochrome was not present in tissue and that there was too little adrenaline available for its formation, recently reported he had proved its presence in saliva gland tissue. He used radioactive tracer techniques which are valuable in metabolic studies.

But it will be a very difficult job to isolate adrenochrome in a pure form. This is not surprising because it is such a reactive chemical—changing so quickly in reaction to other things—that it eludes capture. Special techniques will be required to stabilize it and to extract it. Meanwhile, several research workers have measured adrenochrome and adrenolutin in urine and blood. These were found to be present in higher concentrations in schizophrenic patients.

Professor M. Altschule, Harvard University, Cambridge, Mass., measured adrenolutin levels. He suggested the term "hyperaminochromia" for those mentally ill patients who had increased quantities of adrenolutin in their urine or blood. (Adrenolutin belongs to a class of chemicals called aminochromes.) Dr. E. Kochova in Paris and Prague found adrenochrome in the urine of schizophrenic patients. Professor Altschule and his colleagues have recorded considerable evidence for the presence of adrenochrome, adrenolutin and similar oxidized compounds in the blood. These substances are carried in the blood combined with proteins. The combination is called rheomelanin. The toxic effects of oxygen under pressure (hyperbaric) is due to the excessive formation of these substances.

Other laboratories have added additional information. Drs. B. C. Barrass and D. B. Coult located a substance in the urine of schizophrenic patients which slowed down the destruction of serotonin and at the same time increased the formation of adrenochrome from adrenaline. They suggested that similar enzymes might be present in the brains of schizophrenics and if they were, could cause an increase in serotonin plus an increase in adrenochrome. Either change would be detrimental, but both together would be highly toxic.

Dr. R. Heacock has recently published an excellent account of adrenochrome and adrenolutin.

More recent evidence has finally established that adrenochrome is made in the body in substantial quantities and that most of it is synthesized in heart muscle. Myocardial muscle is very rich in an oxidizing enzyme which changes adrenaline to adrenochrome, noradrenalin to noradrenochrome and other catecholamines to their respective aminochromes. The evidence is now so powerful there is no longer any controversy about the ability of the body to make adrenochrome in vivo.

The new evidence was reviewed by Hoffer in 1985 in the *Journal of Orthomolecular Psychiatry*, vol. 14, pages 262 to 272. Hoffer in 1981 had concluded that the adrenochrome hypothesis accounted for the syndrome of schizophrenia more accurately than did the competing hypotheses. The two main other hypotheses are superfluous since they are inherent in the adrenochrome or more accurately the aminochrome hypothesis. Cadet and Lohr came to the same conclusion in 1987. They wrote, "The dopamine hypothesis has been criticized because it fails to explain many clinical facts and biochemical findings in schizophrenic patients. After a review of the possible neurotoxic effects of free radicals formed during states of high dopamine turnover, we postulate that the neuronal damage caused during these episodes might form the substrate of a comprehensive hypothesis that could potentially explain the protean findings in the group of schizophrenias and the progression of the syndrome, in some patients, to the so-called schizophrenic defect state."

This hypothesis is very interesting for it is essentially what we have been proposing since we first discussed the adrenochrome hypothesis in 1952 before the Dementia Praecox Committee of the Scottish Rites Masons in New York at their meeting in the Canada Room of the Waldorf Astoria Hotel. Apparently Cadet and Lohr are unaware of the large volume of research recorded by our group and others beginning in 1954.

The Presence of Adrenochrome in the Body

As soon as scientists discovered that adrenalin turned pink in solution it appeared likely that what happened so easily in vitro could also occur in the body. Adrenaline is a member of a class of chemicals called catecholamines which polymerize very readily, i.e., they combine with each other to form darkly pigmented compounds with new properties. These new substances are melanins. All the conditions necessary to make these melanins must be present in the body. These are (1) the substrate, the catecholamines, (2) the enzymes which convert these substrata and the trace minerals necessary for this conversion. The oxidation of adrenalin to adrenochrome in water is an example. This requires oxygen and is accelerated by traces of metal such as copper ions. Ideally the final proof would have been the isolation of adrenochrome crystals from blood or other body fluids but because adrenochrome is so unstable it is very difficult to do. Perhaps it could be stabilized by adding semicarbazide to fluids. Adrenochrome semicarbazide is a stable derivative and could be extracted. So far this has not been tried. But nature has already made these stable derivatives, the melanins. The neuromelanins in brain are derived from catecholamines and are easily seen by neuropathologists.

Adrenolutin is a derivative of adrenochrome, just as toxic but causes different psychological changes. It is more stable in blood. Recently a research group in Winnipeg, in the cardiology laboratory of the University of Manitoba, developed a method for measuring how much adrenolutin was present in blood. When they injected adrenalin into rats they were able to show a several fold increase in the amount of adrenolutin in their blood. The amounts found were surprisingly high. The examined the amount of adrenolutin in four species of animals. The values were in rats 0.11 mm/ml, in rabbits 0.08, in dogs 0.05 and in pigs 0.04. From this small series it appears there is a relationship to body size, with the smallest animal having the greatest amount in the blood. This work was reported by Dhalla, Ken S. et al. in *Molecular and Cellular Biochemistry*, 87, 85-92, 1989, under the title "Measurement of adrenolutin as an oxidation product of catecholamines in plasma."

3. REMOVING ADRENOCHROME AND ADRENOLUTIN IS THERAPEUTIC FOR SCHIZOPHRENIA

There are four ways of reducing the amount of adrenochrome and adrenolutin in the body and each one ought to improve schizophrenics if the hypothesis is correct. These are: (1) To reduce the formation of adrenaline; (2) To reduce the formation of adrenochrome; (3) To increase the conversion of adrenochrome into the beneficial compound, dihydroxyindole; (4) To reduce the concentrations of adrenolutin.

Treatments have been developed using each technique, and they have improved the recovery rate of schizophrenics. They will be described briefly in this chapter and in more elaborate detail in the chapter on treatment, Chapter V.

(1) *Reducing production of adrenaline.* There are no effective ways of doing this. By that we mean there are no specific ways. There are many non-specific ways. Since anxiety, conflict, cruelty, bad psychological treatment increase the flow of adrenaline, these should be avoided. Patients should be treated in such a way that adrenaline secretion is reduced, with kindness, understanding and humane treatment.

Certain chemicals may reduce adrenaline levels in one of two ways: by protecting the individual from the impact of external factors or conflicts—these include the barbiturates which help the patient become less aware of anxiety; and by a direct effect on the body—these would include the newer anti-tension compounds such as meprobamate, librium, valium and the more powerful tranquilizers of the phenothiazine class.

We began to use nicotinic acid in 1951 as a treatment for schizophrenia. The results, which have accumulated for nearly twelve years, will be reported in Chapter V. One of the reasons for using nicotinic acid was that theoretically it could reduce the formation of adrenaline by mopping up extra chemicals which the body requires to build it from noradrenaline. There is some slight evidence that this is, in fact, what nicotinic acid does, but more research is required to settle this point.

One might think that removing the adrenal glands would remove all the adrenaline and so prevent adrenochrome from forming. In fact, our early adrenochrome theory was severely condemned by several because removal of both adrenal glands from chronic schizophrenics did not cure them. At that time it was not known that the body could quickly regenerate the tissues which made adrenaline, not in the adrenal gland which is gone, but in other areas of the body. Many tissues can also generate adrenaline. Thus surgery cannot be used to prevent the formation of adrenaline. Nor would we expect chronic patients to be helped even if the adrenaline flow had been interrupted, for there would undoubtedly be permanent changes caused by the disease which would prevent any cure. They can only be improved.

Smoking substantially increases adrenaline secretion. This is due to its nicotine content. Injections of nicotine produce great increases in secretion of adrenaline. For this reason, schizophrenics should be encouraged not to smoke.

(2) *Decreasing production of adrenochrome.* This can be done by using chemicals which decrease the conversion of adrenaline into adrenochrome. We have already discussed the way, by decreasing the amount of adrenaline. But even without changing the concentrations of adrenaline, one might reduce the amount of adrenochrome by taking away those substances needed by adrenaline to facilitate its oxidation, or by making it more difficult for adrenaline to be oxidized.

Substances which could increase the oxidation of adrenaline are copper ions. These are copper atoms which have lost their electrons and are able to float in water. Removing them might be helpful. We have found penicillamine to be one of the best safe compounds which can bind copper and remove it from the body and have, indeed, used it to help us treat schizophrenics in phase three treatment. The second way is to add safe substances such as Vitamin C, ascorbic acid, and glutathione, an amino acid. Both these substances have been found to increase the number of cures in schizophrenia. We use Vitamin C regularly in large doses (3-10 grams per day) to help us treat schizophrenia.

(3) *Decreasing adrenochrome production by converting it into dihydroxyindole.* There would be no point in increasing the production of adrenolutin which is as toxic as adrenochrome. But increasing the concentration of a neutral or anti-tension compound would be helpful. Such a compound is dihydroxyindole which comes from adrenochrome when the body "factory" is functioning normally. If the process of converting adrenochrome into dihydroxyindole instead of adrenolutin could be achieved, the effect would be two-fold; to remove a toxic compound (adrenochrome) and lessen adrenaline's severe effect on the person.

We know of only one way of doing this. This can be done by penicillamine. In the test tube penicillamine combines with adrenochrome and converts most of it into the dihydroxyindole. Thus penicillamine may have two functions, to bind and remove copper and to convert more adrenochrome into the neutral indole.

(4) *Removing adrenolutin.* It may be possible to remove adrenolutin by converting it more rapidly into other non-toxic chemicals, or by mopping it up. We do not know enough about adrenolutin to increase its destruction in this way. But it is possible to mop it up by injecting a substance called ceruloplastmin into the blood. This substance (cp. for short) is normally present in very slight amounts in blood. Much more of it is found in the blood during the last three months of pregnancy, as it is manufactured in the placenta. Cp. binds adrenolutin very firmly and thus removes it from the body. The results of treatment with cp. will be discussed later.

Treatments which one would expect would work if the adrenochrome hypothesis were true, do indeed help patients to recover. We do not wish to imply there are no other treatments, but merely to show that these treatments do work and so the hypothesis is supported.

Malvaria

Research on the adrenochrome-adrenolutin theory has led to the recognition of a disease called "malvaria," which can be diagnosed by a chemical test. Its presence in the majority of untreated schizophrenics. is a fact, not a hypothesis. We have, however, listed malvaria among biochemical theories since it adds much proof to our thesis that biochemical factors play a major role in the production of schizophrenia.

Its history goes back to about five years ago when we expanded the model psychosis hypothesis. Model psychoses are new and strange states of mind produced when normal subjects take compounds such as LSD-25, mescalin, psilocybin, adrenochrome, etc. It is a psychosis, induced by artificial means, which resembles the real psychosis. The "model psychosis hypothesis" is simply the idea that by producing states of severe mental illness in normal subjects, it is possible to learn more about the real psychoses which come on naturally.

We expanded the idea by assuming that the model was active not only in the psychological area but in the biochemical area. That is, that LSD-25 might cause the same changes in the body chemistry that were naturally present in schizophrenia.

Sometime in 1957 our biochemists developed chemical techniques for isolating and demonstrating substances in urine. You can see for yourself how this works when you drop ink on a blotter. If a big blob drops on the blotter, the ink begins to spread from the point from where is was dropped in a radial direction. If you look closely, you can see that there is a clear margin of water which moves faster than the particles of pigment which make up the ink.

In the laboratory, we place a drop of the liquid we want analyzed on specially treated strips of filter paper. The paper is dried and then the strip is dipped in a trough containing specially selected solvents. The liquids, therefore, by a wick action travel up the paper, sweeping along the chemicals which are present in the drop originally placed on the paper. These chemicals travel more slowly than the solvent, just as the particles of ink travel slower than the water, In a certain number of hours, then, they will not have travelled as far on the paper strip as the solvent. How far they travel depends upon the structure of the molecules. Some are swept further from their origin than others and are called fast running or high Rf spots.

After the paper strip has been allowed to stand for eighteen hours, the paper is removed from the trough, dried and sprayed with the chemical which develops it in the same way that a photographic film is developed. The molecules which have moved along the paper react with the spray and produce colored spots. If conditions are ideal, the same molecules always travel to the same area in the paper and given the same color with the spray reagents.

In 1957 we collected urine from alcoholic subjects before and at the height of an LSD-25 experience. We followed the procedure outline above in identifying the chemicals in the specimens. To our pleasure, a mauve-looking spot appeared in the LSD-25 urine sample which had not been present in the sample taken before the drug was administered. We then collected a small series of urine samples from schizophrenic and normal subjects and had them analyzed in the same way. All the schizophrenics showed the same spot. None of the other subjects tested did. This began our series of extensive studies which have been carried out at four of our research laboratories in Saskatchewan. The spot was called any one of the following names: mauve spot, unidentified substances or u.s. for short.

Since then over one thousand patients have been examined for the absence or presence of the mauve factor. A detailed report will not be given here since the data has been reported in the psychiatric literature. The following table shows the proportions of various groups according to diagnosis who have the mauve factor.

Schizophrenics untreated and ill less than one year have the greatest incidence of subjects with mauve factor in the urine. Normal subjects have none.

Since a small proportion of schizophrenic subjects do not have the mauve factor and small proportions of the other groups do, it was not possible to use the presence of mauve factor as a diagnostic test for schizophrenia. This is not surprising for it is generally true that diagnosis in psychiatry, while as precise as diagnosis in other branches of medicine which have no laboratory tests, is not precise enough to guarantee that every patient labelled schizophrenic is in fact schizophrenic, and every person not labelled schizophrenic, is not. Furthermore, it is possible that some patients with clinical schizophrenia have other biochemical abnormalities not measured by the mauve test.

DIAGNOSIS	NUMBER EXAMINED	PER CENT WHO HAVE FACTOR
A. *Normal subjects*	60	0
B. *Subjects physically ill*		
1. Adults	100	10
2. Children	100	10
C. *Neurotic subjects*	200	20
D. *Alcoholics*	40	40
E. *Schizophrenics*		
1. No treatment at any time and illness present less than one year	100	75
2. Treated successfully	40	0
3. Treated unsuccessfully (mostly chronic patients from mental hospital)	200	50
F. *Mental retardation*		
1. Physically normal	20	50
2. Physically abnormal	20	0
G. *Alcoholics after LSD*	40	35

For these and other reasons we decided to use the mauve test as the main diagnostic laboratory test in much the same way as the Wassermann test is used for syphilis. As a result, we decided that every human who had mauve factor in the urine had a disease called malvaria, regardless of any other diagnosis given him by other diagnosticians. This was an operational definition depending entirely on the chemical test. A verbal definition is a series of statements about something. These are found in dictionaries. But the accuracy of the definition depends upon the meaning of other words and there is much room for argument.

An operational definition is a definition which depends, not upon other words, but upon a series of accurately described procedures which any trained person can follow and reproduce. In this case, any chemist who follows the written instructions, can show when the mauve factor is present in urine. Thus, the area of disagreement about whether the mauve factor is present or not is sharply reduced.

Malvaria, then, is that disease which is present in any human being when he excretes a mauve factor. Thus, there can no longer be any argument about malvaria. It is, or is not, present, and the decision is made by the chemical test.

But does it have any use in the practice of psychiatry and in the care of the mentally ill? Malvaria would be a meaningless term unless it turned out that having malvaria leads to proper specific treatment. The only objective of diagnosis is to determine treatment and to establish prognosis... the future of the disease. In other words, is it of any help to know that a subject has malvaria? How is the patient with malvaria different than the patient who does not have it?

The problem has been examined in the following ways:

(1) By examining large groups of patients of all diagnostic classes to find out what malvarians, regardless of diagnosis, have in common with one another.
(2) By giving malvarians and non-malvarians a series of psychological tests for comparison.
(3) By giving the two groups a series of physiological tests for comparison.
(4) By examining the group of malvarians and non-malvarians not treated with nicotinic acid or nicotinamide for response to treatment and prognosis.
(5) By examining the group of malvarians and non-malvarians which were treated with nicotinic acid for response to treatment and prognosis.
(6) By comparing malvarians and non-malvarians for psychological response to LSD-25.

The results of these large-scale studies are as follows:

(1) Are malvarians different clinically from non-malvarians? The answer is "yes." We have compared 104 malvarians, with 75 subjects who did not have malvaria, drawn at random from a group of 150 non-malvarians.

Whether they were diagnosed schizophrenic, neurotic, or neither of these, patients whose urine tests showed the mauve factor were more like each other than patients whose urine did not. Even non-malvarians who were schizophrenic seldom had the vivid perceptual changes of the schizophrenics who also had malvaria.

In general, malvarians have a much higher incidence of

perceptual changes. They more frequently show disturbances in thought content and the process of thinking is disturbed. They show inappropriate mood changes much more frequently and bizarre and unusual changes in behavior. The only symptom which was present as frequently in both groups of patients was depression or low spirits.

(2) Were malvarians and non-malvarians psychologically different? Yes. When examined with the HOD test, malvarians scored nearly twice as high. They scored higher on the Minnesota Multiphasic Test. When examined for certain visual tests which measure constance of perception, they showed more rigidity. The differences were large and statistically significant.

(3) Were malvarians and non-malvarians physiologically different? Examination of certain changes in brain wave patterns showed malvarians had more abnormality than non-malvarians.

(4) What difference was there in response to treatment and prognosis of the two groups not treated with nicotinic acid or nicotinamide? Ordinary psychiatric treatment produced different results in the two groups. In general, patients with malvaria (whether they were neurotic or psychotic) did not respond as well to treatment, had to stay in hospital longer for treatment, and needed to be re-admitted more often after discharge.

(5) What difference was there when nicotinic acid was used in treatment? When nicotinic acid was included in the treatment program, those with malvaria began to recover much sooner, much better and in larger numbers than non-malvarians (the methods will be described later).

This applied to all diagnostic groups, the mentally retarded, adolescent problems, anxiety neuroses, alcoholics and schizophrenics. For example, six malvarian alcoholics were treated with LSD-25 as a main treatment. They were not improved whatever and are still alcoholic. But out of eight alcoholic malvarians treated with nicotinic acid, seven have been sober over two years each.

Non-malvarians do not respond nearly as well to nicotinic acid. In the past three years we have given nicotinamide treatment to seven children with malvaria and twenty without it. All were either afflicted with behavioral problems or were unable to learn in school.

Of the seven with malvaria, six are nearly well and getting on well. The seventh, a child of one year of age, was treated for only one month while expecting admission to a school for mentally defective children. After admission, the vitamin was no longer given and there was no improvement. Of the twenty non-malvarian children, only one has shown any improvement of significance.

(6) Do malvarians and non-malvarians respond differently psychologically to LSD-25? Yes. Out of any group of normal subjects given LSD-25, about one-half will have an experience which we term "psychedelic." That is, they are relaxed, at ease, and have exciting and useful experiences, many times of a mystical or visionary sort from which they derive lasting benefit.

Alcoholics without malvaria show the same incidence; about half will have these psychedelic reactions. This type of reaction seems to be important to treatment. Several of our workers have observed that alcoholics who do have these good experiences provide the majority of recoveries.

However, alcoholics who have malvaria, either before or after the LSD-25 session, are different. Less than one-fifth have relaxed and good experiences and hardly any have a deep visionary, religious or other experience.

This evidence, collected over a two-year period, shows the usefulness of the diagnosis of malvaria. The presence of the mauve factor indicates that the patients are seriously ill and should be given nicotinic acid treatment as well as other treatments. It allows one to predict that if they are given such treatment, the results will be much better than if they are not.

Finally, if the mauve factor vanishes from the urine, it is a hopeful sign that the patients are beginning to recover. So far, no patient who has recovered has remained malvarian. In addition, a recurrence of the malvaria is a bad prognostic sign and suggests that active treatment should be instituted right away.

Dr. Irvine and his coworkers established the structure of the mauve factor. It is kryptopyrrole (KP), a well-known chemical. This work has been confirmed by A. Sohler, R. Beck and J. J. Noval, who first demonstrated that it produced behavioral changes in animals. This work has been expanded by Dr. K. Krischer and Dr. Carl C. Pfeiffer who suggested that both KP and a nicotinic schizophrenic sweat factor came from a common precursor. Pfeiffer found that KP bound with pyridoxine (vitamin

B-6) and could therefore produce a vitamin B-6 deficiency. He therefore suggested that the presence of the mauve factor (KP) is an indication for giving increased quantities of vitamin B-6 to patients.

The Serotonin Hypothesis

Serotonin is an indole ultimately derived from the amino-acid, tryptophane. Tryptophane is an interesting substance found in the brain, the gut, the platelets (small particles in the blood which break up and help form clots to decrease bleeding), and in some other organs or tissues of the body. It is one of the building blocks for proteins. Since the body cannot manufacture it, it must come from food. Without it, the body develops lack of growth and other pathological changes.

If a chunk of muscle is taken from an organ, kept in a special solution and attached to a pen, there will be tracings on a moving strip of paper when it contracts. If LSD-25 is placed on top of this muscle strip, the substance will make the muscle contract. But if the muscle is pre-treated with serotonin, there will no longer be a reaction.

This observation (and others) led D. W. Woolley to suggest that some forms of mental disease might be due to disturbance in the way serotonin is used in the brain. The reasoning then was that since serotonin worked against LSD-25, the action of the drug was made possible by some interference in normal serotonin activity. Woolley proposed that either too little or too much serotonin might be responsible chemically for schizophrenia.

Dr. Woolley was a co-discoverer of the fact that nicotinic acid is a vitamin. He is now on the staff of the Rockefeller Institute for Medical Research in New York City. In spite of his near blindness he has continued to do stimulating and creative research. He was one of the first scientists to focus biochemical attention in a rational way to the problems of mental disease. He was rudely told by some world-famous psychiatrists to mind his own business, but luckily he continued to examine, for his business was to examine the operations of mind from the point of view of the biochemist.

His serotonin idea spurred on a tremendous amount of research. It was supported by certain other findings, for example, that some tranquilizers and some anti-depressants caused the levels of serotonin to rise and fall, and at the same time certain changes in behavior were seen. The final point of evidence in favor of the idea was the fact that serotonin had been extracted from tissues and was believed to be present in the brain. There was therefore no disagreement about serotonin's existence.

Against the hypothesis were many arguments. For one thing, the levels of serotonin in biological fluids had no relationship to mental disease. None of the products known to come from serotonin was related to mental disease. When injected in the body, serotonin produced no changes of the kind produced by LSD-25 or adrenochrome. No newer therapies for schizophrenia have resulted from this theory. Finally, the theory is not satisfactory for the clinical psychiatrist for it does not account for the emotions and therefore does not allow them to play a role, nor does it account for many of the physical and mental changes found in schizophrenia. It will be shown later that the adrenochrome hypothesis does account for many of these factors in a simple and economical way. In other words, as we pointed out earlier, the serotonin theory does not account for the disease in any satisfactory way.

However, it is no weaker or stronger than the acetylocholine theory. Acetylocholine appears to be a neurohormone which has something to do with the transmission of stimuli or messages in the brain. Too little or too much can produce marked changes in brain operation. But this is also true of any brain constituent, including sodium, potassium, cholesterol, sugar, and others.

Psychological Factors (contributing causes)

Psychological theories generally ignore biochemical factors or minimize them as signs of stress or of the schizophrenia. We will not attempt to discuss all the psychological theories which have been proposed for they are too numerous, poorly formulated and not well based upon evidence of a scientific nature, and many of their originators have themselves been very dubious about their value.

Freud once claimed that analysts must do their work very quickly before the physicians came along with their syringes. He later changed his mind about his own theories, and thought at one time mental illness might have a biochemical basis. Harry Stack Sullivan, a famous psychiatrist known for his work on schizophrenia, and Adolf Meyer, another psychiatrist who claimed everything was important in the patient's history or everyday life, were two of the strongest advocates of the use of psychology in treatment of the mentally ill. But even they, like most of the early enthusiastic psychoanalytic advocates, used many escape clauses in their writings, in inconspicuous ways, of course, like the small, unreadable print in some contracts.

Because he did not understand the natural phenomena he witnessed in mental illness, Freud filled the mind with small creatures, just as primitive man, who did not understand sun, moon, thunder and lightning, peopled the sky with gods. Freud called his small mind creatures the Id, the Ego and the Superego, and he imagined them as not being able to get along with one another.

What is completely amazing is that these ideas should have received such wide acceptance in North America by well-educated people, when the data which has slowly accumulated has usually contradicted these theories. This must be a tribute to Freud's great ability as a writer (he was once considered for the Nobel prize in literature).

All psychological theories of schizophrenia are basically variants of the same theme based upon psychoanalytic doctrine, that the mother (or father, or both) is to blame for the child's schizophrenia. Followers of this idea cling to it so tenaciously that one is tempted to wonder if they go into the profession because they hate their mothers (or fathers).

The doctrine claims that a defect develops in the mother-infant or mother-child relationship, usually because there is some imperfection in the mother. As a result, the child does not develop in a normal way and later on, when life becomes more difficult and demanding, the subject retires into a world of fantasy or unreality which he finds more pleasant than the real world. There is a basic personality defect at the root of the illness and until this is remedied, we are told, there can be no true and lasting cure. Only analysis can bring about such a permanent change in personality and so cure the patient.

The symptoms and signs which are present are considered to be projections or wish fulfillments and result from conflicts induced by the bad mothering from which the child suffered. Symptoms like hallucinations are considered to be projections of sub-conscious wishes and symptoms like paranoid delusions are believed to represent homosexual fears.

The theory of subconscious projection of wishes or fantasies cannot be seriously examined for there is no way of knowing what is going on in the subconscious. Psychoanalysts consider their method, free association and dreams, the royal road to the unconscious. The trouble is that words have so many meanings, any interpretation can be given to the random utterances of disturbed people. There has been no advance whatever in the theory of interpretation of dreams since Freud. To some, the interpretation of dreams is just as scientific as examining the entrails of chickens or reading tea leaves. Too much is left to the imagination of the interpreter.

There is precious little evidence that homosexual fears lead to paranoias. The original idea was based upon one patient's account, High Court Judge Schreber, who feared that he was being changed into a woman, i.e., that he would be deprived of his sexual organs. It is difficult to understand why this was interpreted as a homosexual panic. Homosexuality refers to sex relations between members of the same sex. Did Schreber wish to be a male homosexual and so not wish to become a female; or did he wish to become a female homosexual, and finding this wish repugnant, repudiate it by having paranoid ideas? The evidence today is no stronger than it was seventy years ago. In fact, if Freud were to come back today, he would find very little which is new in psychoanalysis.

It seems to have been forgotten that Schreber's "homosexual fears," which have been made so much of, were among many symptoms. Schreber, who wrote a very clear and excellent account of his illness, had a vast number of other strange experiences. The fear of being changed into a woman was only one of many hundreds of queer happenings which he reported, including the hallucination of the grand piano in his room.

In general, schizophrenics lose their sexual drives or find them reduced in intensity while ill. But the incidence of homosexuality either before, during or after the illness, is no greater among schizophrenics than among normal subjects. One would expect that there would be a high degree of homosexuality among schizophrenics locked up together in large wards in mental hospitals, but it seems likely homosexuality is far more rampant in prisons, armies, ships at sea and in residential schools than in wards of mental hospitals.

We will propose another kind of psychological theory which may be called the perceptual theory of schizophrenia. This theory, combined with the biochemical theories, allows one to account economically (without bringing in ideas which cannot be tested) for most of the symptomatology.

Our basic assumption is that the biochemical changes somehow interfere with normal perception. As a result the external world is seen, heard, etc. in an unusual or distorted way. The subject is unaware the change has occurred in him and believes it has occurred in the environment. He therefore reacts appropriately to what he perceives in the new world, but to the observer his actions are inappropriate.

An example may illustrate what we mean. In normal use, certain figures are punched on the keyboard of an ordinary calculator in certain order. This is the data or information which is fed in from the environment. Then the machine performs certain operations such as adding and multiplying. The final result appears as an answer on strips of paper, or on certain dials.

As long as the correct data is punched in, and the machine performs its operations accurately, the result will be satisfactory. Suppose, however, the machine begins to produce a series of random answers, some right, some wrong. The error may lie in the data punched in, or in the way the data was punched in. Or the data fed in may be handled incorrectly because of some defect in the machine. Then the answers are bound to be wrong.

The same reasoning can apply to a human being. A human being is normal as long as the information from the environment is received in the usual stable way, is used by him in the expected manner and is acted upon in a rational way. A failure in any one of these three facets of normality can produce irrational behavior. The three mechanisms are perception, thought and action. In our theory, disorders of perception plus disorders in thinking can account for the final disorder we know as schizophrenia.

We will provide the evidence which supports this theory. Before doing so, however, we should point out that one of the early physicians to enunciate a perceptual hypothesis was Thomas Willis, who stated over three hundred years ago that psychotic patients seemed to see the world through a distorted looking glass. John Conolly, the eminent English psychiatrist, and his colleagues Pinel and Rush, had a well-developed perceptual theory over one hundred years ago. Conolly stated that many patients rolled on the floor because their skin was too warm and that patients believed their food was poisoned because it had a coppery taste.

Evidence for the Perceptual Theory in Schizophrenia

Perceptual changes are present in the majority of schizophrenic patients. This has already been discussed in detail in Chapter II. Any psychiatrist who wishes to corroborate this needs only to spend some time taking a careful history of all the possible perceptual changes.

A useful guide is the HOD test. This test is based to a large degree on the presence of perceptual changes. It includes 145 cards, and the patient is asked to sort these into two piles, true and false. If the subject has a significant number of true answers, he is usually considered to be ill. The test was developed by the authors in 1961 on the basis of differences we had observed between people who had schizophrenia and those who did not. It was correlated with the mauve factor test and it was found that most subjects scoring high on the test also had the mauve factor. It was, therefore, a diagnostic test for malvaria as well as for schizophrenia.

From the answers given as true, it was possible for us to form a picture of the group of patients who are malvarian. We found that as a group, they believed that people were watching them more than they had done in the past, and in fact watched them all the time. They have visions of people when their eyes are closed. They feel unreal and see others as unreal. There is a mist or fog shutting them away from the world. Many times objects and people, as well as their own faces, look strange and therefore they misidentify people. Often they see sparks of light or spots floating before them and the world may suddenly look dim. They have out-of-the-body experiences.

The accounts by recovered schizophrenic patients of their own illnesses are rich in perceptual changes. One patient said that her feet looked queer and small and things looked bright and glared. Another saw her hands, feet, neck and part of her face swollen.

One patient experienced a visionary state. The hand of his

enemy descended upon his arm which caused his hand to become white. His brain opened and a message was tapped out by his enemy which was slanderous and threatening. He became frightened, left his farm and moved to a hotel where he lived for eight months before admission.

A 51-year-old woman came to hospital in response to a voice which told her to. Two weeks before admission she had visual hallucinations of a mouse, which seemed to say "Judas" to her, moving on the curtains. She also believed she was being influenced by hypnosis.

For another patient, people seemed far away, everything appeared to float away from her and her head appeared large and floating above her body.

The chief complaint of one patient was dizziness, numbness and quivery feelings; print danced up and down before her, when she was lying down the bed moved under her, turning quickly made her dizzy and once her arm felt bigger and wider.

One 52-year-old patient heard voices telling him his psychiatrist would kill him and so he was afraid to sleep at night.

A 24-year-old girl believed her husband or some external agency controlled her in an unusual way.

These symptoms were usually accompanied by others... suspiciousness, incoherence of speech, delusions, gross thought disorder. Some had hallucinations of two or three of the sense organs. Many were depressed and anxious.

We found that patients with schizophrenia feel better when they can discuss their symptoms with friends who had also had schizophrenia. Schizophrenic patients who are allowed to discuss their perceptual changes will very often accept them as a rational explanation for their difficulties. One of our patients developed an increased sensitivity to odors. He was a farmer and, unaware that he had changed, he assumed that the barn was too dirty and needed to be cleaned. He began a series of maneuvers to clean his barn including extraordinary cleansing procedures, with deodorants and ventilating systems. When it was suggested to him that his sense of smell had become overly sensitive he looked surprised. He accepted the explanation and immediately ceased his activities.

Objective tests have shown that schizophrenics have a rigid kind of visual perception which prevents them from stabilizing their external world. Objects appear usually too small and perspective is altered. When a schizophrenic is looked at, he often believes people are looking directly at him when, in fact, they are looking beyond him, to his left or to his right.

Perceptual changes can be induced in normal subjects by hypnosis, bringing about symptoms resembling those of schizophrenia. This can be done during the trance or in the post-trance state, providing a method for giving subjects perceptual changes while they are hypnotized and allowing these changes to continue after the hypnosis. This makes it possible to study the reaction of these subjects to other people about them.

A large series of experiments of this kind were carried out by Dr. S. Fogel and Dr. A. Hoffer in Saskatoon on two normal subjects who were trained in becoming hypnotized. After they had achieved a deep trance state, certain changes were induced by command, "When you come out of your trance you will find that (here the key suggestion was given). When I snap my finger you will be normal again." The suggestions covered all the perceptual areas including time, for example, "You will find that people are watching you," "People's faces look funny," "Everything looks blue," or "Time is moving very quickly."

During the experiments we observed the following results:

Visual perceptual changes. At the command, "You will find people are watching you," the subjects developed a typical, even exaggerated clinical picture of paranoid schizophrenia. They were hostile, suspicious, irritable, and difficult. On one occasion a subject was taken to be interviewed by a psychiatrist who did not know she was in the post-trance state. At no time during hypnosis was the subject given the suggestion to become schizophrenic or paranoid, yet twenty minutes after the interview began the psychiatrist was preparing to write out committal papers to send her to a mental hospital.

In this post-trance state she vehemently denied she had been hypnotized or that people were not watching her. This paranoid reaction was easily demonstrated in the presence of one or more observers, and on one occasion it was demonstrated to the research meeting of the College of Medicine, University of Saskatchewan.

We produced emotional reactions to visual changes, which resembled the behavior of schizophrenics. In one experiment, the subject was told that all colors would be alike. She thereupon became sad and depressed, and had visual hallucinations. Disorientation to her environment was complete. The suggestion that all colors were bright, on the other hand, produced manic behavior. She was happy, excited, spoke rapidly and was very gay. She read and walked more quickly than usual and laughed easily. Again she was completely disoriented.

The feeling that there was no color anywhere, suggested during hypnosis, produced hostility, suspiciousness, depression and irritability. When told that she would not be able to recognize anyone in the room but herself and the hypnotizer, the subject became suspicious of everyone except the hypnotizer. She demanded to see Dr. Hoffer's credentials before acknowledging him as a doctor. She thought Dr. Hoffer's metronome was a time bomb and, had it not been for her faith in the hypnotizer, she would have run away.

Upon being told that everyone present was sinister, she became suspicious, hostile, argumentative, sarcastic, insulting and belligerent.

Changes in hearing. The subjects' reactions to suggested changes in hearing followed the same pattern. One subject heard voices and became suspicious and hostile when told that all sounds would be louder. But when told that all sounds would be quieter, she became depressed, unhappy, quiet and withdrawn. The suggestion that she would not be able to locate the source of any sound she heard produced another interesting response. She withdrew and became silent, refusing to answer any questions. When we insisted, she folded both arms over her face and withdrew into herself in a peculiar way as if to shut out all sight and sound.

Changes in smell. We were able to produce similar changes when we told the subject that all odors would be exaggerated. She said her name was Rose, which it was not, and became angry and unfriendly. She said she could smell the pond in a picture we showed her, and she believed she could actually get into the cold water. She was very argumentative and resented questioning. But when told she had no sense of smell at all, she presented a pathetic, childlike picture of bewilderment, worry and confusion. She became withdrawn and vague.

Changes in touch. We suggested to the subject that her sense of touch would be heightened. As a result, she became possessive about a linen handkerchief that was handed to her and refused to give it up as she continued to feel it with her fingers. She was not interested in a dry sponge or other coarse objects, but smooth objects occupied her full attention. She was distant and not as communicative as usual. She was then told she would not be able to feel anything. She thereupon became hostile and scornful and said her name was Susie, which it was not. She was again suspicious and argumentative, aggressive and angry, a typical paranoid schizophrenic.

Changes in time perception. For these experiments we used a metronome which has a loud regular beat and which could be adjusted in frequency from 0 to several hundred beats a minute. The subjects were hypnotized and the frequency, to begin with, was set at sixty beats a minute. The subjects were then given the suggestion, "When you come out of your trance, you will find the clock beating sixty beats a minute." Then the subjects were ordered to come out of the trance.

At this point, they appeared little altered. When the frequency was decreased to thirty beats a minute without their knowledge, however, they were markedly slowed up. They thought slowly and acted slowly, said they were depressed and appeared to be depressed.

When the beat was stopped, the subjects became catatonic almost immediately, literally stopped in their tracks, even if they were walking rapidly or engaged in any activity at the time. One subject developed a typical waxy flexibility. When she was placed in any position she seemed frozen in it indefinitely. The other developed a rigid negativistic catatonia from which she could not be moved. When the beat was started again they both resumed their activity as if there had been no pause at all. In fact, they vigorously denied they had stopped or paused or interrupted what they were doing, in any way.

When the beat was set to exceed sixty a minute, the subjects became more alert, more friendly and more active. They spoke more rapidly, stated that they felt wonderful and appeared to be hypomanic.

We will not give the details of all the experiments. We can, however, say that they proved that when normal subjects were exposed to perceptual changes, and when they accepted them as real, their behavior was abnormal and reproduced the varieties of schizophrenia seen clinically. It was possible, by giving the appropriate perceptual change, to demonstrate nearly every variety of schizophrenia, including hebephrenia, catatonia, paranoia and the simple forms.

Dr. B. Aaronsen, at the New Jersey Bureau of Research in Neurology and Psychiatry, has corroborated our work and expanded it into new and exciting dimensions. He has shown that profound changes in behavior are produced by these techniques, as well as major changes in responses to the Minnesota Multiphasic Personality Inventory (MMPI) test.

The evidence, then, is fairly strong that perceptual changes, if accepted as true by the patients, will produce bizarre and abnormal behavior. The readers can, as an exercise, imagine what these perceptual changes would do to him. Let him suppose that people are watching him all the time, or that his face in the mirror seems strange or that he cannot tell where sounds are coming from. We are sure this small exercise would be very enlightening.

Further research will determine how important these changes are in determining the content of the schizophrenic illness.

Sociological Factors

By these we mean interaction of the schizophrenic person with people about him. This is a vast subject and we will illustrate tiny portions of it. Our basic hypothesis is that changes in perception will determine this interaction. An example is the baby's reaction to mother. There is, undoubtedly, in schizophrenia some pathology in the relationship, but it is more likely present in the sick child.

One of the first interactions between mothers and child is the smile. It does not matter much who smiles first, mother or child. Usually the other responds, perhaps involuntarily, and a mutual interaction is developed.

Suppose, because of some perceptual difficulty, the baby does not recognize the mother's smile as a smile, and from the beginning there is no bond or interaction. It is not difficult to imagine how hard it would be for mother to continue to do all the things she must do without getting an appropriate response from the child.

Suppose a child at the age of six months has a disorder of

hearing and cannot tell where sounds are coming from. When his mother talks to him, he sees her, but the sound of her voice comes from somewhere else. He, therefore, cannot associate mother's voice with mother and so does not respond to her. Her voice then has no more significance to him than the ticking of the clock, the radio, or the refrigerator. This kind of change could explain why mothers of such children believe that their children are deaf.

Let us assume that an adult schizophrenic develops a disorder in the perception of time, so that time is moving more slowly for him. Imagine what it might be like to hold a conversation with him. When a statement is made, the patient should respond in a time interval which we would consider normal to him. But since his sense of time is slow, he would respond to the normal person only after a prolonged pause. But subjects would, therefore, be out of step with respect to their own conceptions of time. The normal subject might become impatient and repeat his statement before the patient could reply, and in a louder voice. The patient might then wonder why the other person raised his voice or spoke so quickly to him.

Or imagine what would happen if a schizophrenic patient could no longer judge how loud he would have to speak to project his voice to another person. He might speak so loudly, not knowing he was doing so, that he would irritate everyone about him. If people pointed out to him that his voice was too loud he might not believe them and become hostile and suspicious.

With these handicaps, the patient would be less able to pick up all the cues of normal social intercourse which are so important. He would be placed at a tremendous disadvantage and would have to decide intellectually how to act in the absence of these cues. This would be difficult for he would have to know first what is wrong, and even then he would be unaware of much that happens because he would assume it was perfectly natural.

We have seen many patients whose entire bizarre behavior was readily accounted for by a few perceptual changes. One was a school teacher whose hearing became so acute he could hear people talking several rooms away from him. Another patient found that he could not distinguish one face from another and, therefore, concluded the same person was everywhere and following him about.

Schizophrenics will talk to their hallucinations and hold conversations with them. They may even follow imaginary instructions; many patients will refuse to eat because their stomachs feel dead or they taste something bitter and assume they are being poisoned. Disorders of smell can lead them to believe they are being gassed.

With the perceptual hypothesis of schizophrenia, it is no longer necessary to consider that the schizophrenic is the most obvious symptom of a sick family. There is little doubt that a schizophrenic member of a family could easily disrupt the entire family relationships, especially if the family is unaware he is sick. For they would find the patient responding in unusual and inappropriate ways to their attempts to interact normally with him.

This has led some sociologists to place the cart before the horse, and to blame the family for producing the schizophrenia in the sick member. Recently a paper was published in a psychiatric journal in which the author claimed that many mothers deliberately made their children schizophrenic in order to satisfy some deep-routed complex of their own. This idea is no more fantastic than many similar purely psychological or sociological ideas.

We have seen many so-called "schizophrenic" families with schizophrenic mothers. The families were tense, unhappy, hostile. Yet when the patient returned home cured, the same family became normal and mother no longer seemed so pathological. Because, strange as it may seem, mothers and fathers too are human and make mistakes, and become distressed when their children are sick. When they are anxious and upset, they do not always behave as wisely or as kindly as one would hope. However, we have found many relatives of schizophrenic patients to be devoted to them and to have helped them enormously. Not all relatives of schizophrenics are amiable paragons of virtue, and in this respect they resemble the rest of us. But considering how badly informed they often are, in our experience they do as well as anyone could expect.

CHAPTER IV

COMPREHENSIVE THEORY OF SCHIZOPHRENIA

A SCIENTIFIC theory can be compared to a building. A building must have a foundation. Similarly, a scientific theory is built upon a foundation of facts available from all the research which has been completed at the time it is created. It then grows and develops with further research as new facts are accumulated and old ones expanded.

A theory has two important functions. The first is to provide a logical and intellectually satisfying explanation for the facts which make up the problem. If this is not done, we will have a problem which is not related to the theory. And facts divorced of their proper theory are as incomplete as the pile of bricks from which the house will be built.

The second function is to provide a guide for further exploration and research. If this is done, it will have led the research into previously unexplored territories, yielding valuable and sometimes undreamed-of information. These new facts will mold the theory as research progresses until in its final form, it is unrecognizable. Thus, theories, when research is completed, often have as little resemblance to the original supposition as houses have to the foundations on which they are built.

For theories live only to be altered, and any theory which survives too long unchanged, has become fossilized by the veneration of dogma or the scientific incompetence of its disciples. This is what has happened to the psychoanalytic theory.

The theory we will present of schizophrenia is, like most living theories, incomplete, and more work must and will be done on it. It is based upon evidence reported in scientific journals and books, which we think are accumulated by the best research. It is, therefore, the best we have been able to put together, so far.

It remains to this day the only theory which has attempted, and in our opinion has succeeded, in accounting for most of the biological, psychological and sociological vagaries which occur in this illness. Other theories have either ignored bodily peculiarities found in schizophrenia, or else have made little or no attempt to relate these peculiarities to the psychological and sociological disturbances, considering them to be no more important than the waving of blades of grass in the wind.

We hope, indeed, that our theories will be out of date very quickly as evidence about schizophrenia continues to accumulate. In our own continued researches we will do our best to make them obsolete.

We will not give references for each point of our theory as we would if this book was meant to be read only by scientists, since we wish to present it as simply as possible, in an interesting and accurate way, not only to medical men and researchers, but also to people who know little about schizophrenia except from having lived in, or alongside it.

Finally, we do not claim that our theory is the only true one, nor that it is accepted by our colleagues. The theory is not generally accepted, nor even widely known, and there are many who will find it completely abhorrent. This is their right. We hope they will debate it with us, objectively, on the basis of facts and in only one forum—the scientific press.

We will first outline our comprehensive theory, and then describe five cases: (1) in infancy, (2) in adolescence, (3) during maturity in a woman, (4) during maturity in a man, and (5) during old age.

These are not case histories about individual patients, but the experiences of many patients which have been combined and condensed for the sake of clarity and better understanding of what can, and does, happen when schizophrenia comes on during these periods of life.

Our comprehensive theory of schizophrenia may be summarized as follows:

> Due to chromosomes (which contain genes) derived parents, the person uses normal chemicals in an abnormal way.

2. As a result, at a certain time in life toxic chemicals are produced in the body which interfere with the normal operations of brain and body.

3. Therefore, the world and the body as experienced by all the senses appears to be altered—strange, different, unreal, etc.

4. But the person has learned to accept the evidence of the senses as real or true, and continues to do so. He is unaware the changes are due to changes in his brain and believes it is the world external to him which is altered.

5. He reacts in a way he considers appropriate, but as the perceptions are inappropriate so must be his actions as judged by others. If many people, or even society, lived in similar worlds they would react in similar ways.

6. His total behavior personality, etc. is, therefore, different and this brings into play a host of social consequences in family, friends, society, etc.

7. This results in action by society which may place him in hospital, in jail or banish him to a neighboring country.

Inheritance

The many notable studies of Professor Franz Kallman, Professor Eliot Slater, Professor Erik Stromgren and many others have shown that a tendency to schizophrenia is inherited. Their conclusions have survived twenty-five years of harsh criticisms and are now well enough established to have been publicly endorsed by Professor Paul Meehl, president of the American Psychological Association.

There are still those, however, who doubt that schizophrenia is a physical inherited disease, and most of these seem to have failed to recognize the significance of a well-known fact, that the disease occurs in about one per cent of the human race. It has never been explained by these sceptics why an illness, often thought to be due to an unfitness of its sufferers for the full rigors of life, should occur in so many people.

Two recent publications firmly establish the genetic basis of schizophrenia. The first by Kety, Rosenthal, Wender and Schulsinger (1968) is a general review of the nature-nurture debate and comes out positive for the biological nature, while

Gottesman and Shields' (1972) fine volume, using twins as a basis, conclude that specific genetic factors clearly underlie schizophrenia, whereas environmental factors are nonspecific and idiosyncratic. Schizophrenia they described as the "outcome of a genetically determined developmental predisposition."

It is also generally not admitted, although it is well known, that the illness itself confers physical advantages on its victims. Dr. J. Lucy showed that schizophrenics have an extraordinary tolerance for injected histamine. Lea demonstrated that schizophrenic soldiers have a very low incidence of allergies compared with similar young soldiers who have had head injuries.

Rheumatoid arthritis is a very infrequent occurrence among schizophrenics. Ehrentheil's studies suggest that they are not as likely to suffer shock after such catastrophies as the perforation of an internal organ, or a coronary thrombosis. Our own enquiry shows that they are highly resistant to wound and surgical shock after grave injuries and burns.

This superiority may seem a high price to pay for a tendency to a disease like schizophrenia, but for some people it may be of vital importance to survival. To hunters and food gatherers, for example, allergy could be a matter of life or death. A hunter who is allergic to pollens might not be able to hunt and so would expose himself and his family to the danger of starvation. If he became partly blinded and deafened by hay fever, he might himself become the victim of another predator.

If injured, he would have a higher resistance to wound shock. If lost, he could stand cold and privation better than others. Like many schizophrenics, he might well survive misfortunes which would kill his fellows.

His perceptual difficulties, or even frank hallucinations, might cause him little or no distress. Like most hunters and food gatherers, he would be living in a very small, tightly knit society isolated from settled areas, where communication is lacking, mutual support is essential and tolerance is high. For his counterpart in a more populated farm or city area, the same psychological changes might be far more disruptive, and have serious social consequences.

In fact, these changes may work to his advantage, for the ability to see visions and endure various hardships is highly esteemed among many hunting people. Not only does this bind the group together, but it enhances the prestige of those who are favored in this manner. Far from being despised, outcast or persecuted, they can become valued members of society whose gifts are highly regarded and used for the common good. They are likely to have special duties which might not only reduce their chances of being killed while hunting, but increase their chances of breeding.

A close look at history shows that those whose perceptions ranged from the unusual to the bizarre have, from time to time, had great influence on art, politics, philosophy, religion and science, greatly altering not only the viewpoint but the actions of our whole species.

Schizophrenia, then, appears to be beneficial as well as harmful to the individual and to the species, and can be useful to man if properly understood. A careful study of the genetics and biochemical nature of the disease will help us obtain not only an increased knowledge of a great illness, but a better understanding of those life-saving qualities with which it seems to be associated.

Even if we wish to ignore these facts, however, the remarkable twin studies of Kallman and Slater are absolutely convincing in themselves. Recently their work was confirmed in a most unlikely way when four girls, quadruplets, developed schizophrenia within a few years of each other. Their case was described by David Rosenthal.

The quadruplets were studied in extraordinary detail by a team of over twenty-four investigators supported by the National Institute of Mental Health of the U.S. government, in Washington, D.C. It was found that all four girls and their father had the same kind of brain wave electrical patterns. All four developed a similar kind of schizophrenia and it unfolded in the same manner. All four were underactive, had difficulty talking, were depressed and socially isolated. A grandmother was psychotic. The father had unreasonable, out-of-place rages and a life-long pattern of secrecy and lying. The investigators, therefore, concluded that the girls' illnesses were understandable in terms of a combination of inherited and environmental factors.

The inheritance factor helps us to explain why some members of a family are schizophrenic and some are not. The person likely to become schizophrenic inherits from his parents a number of genes for schizophrenia which make possible the biochemical processes which we will describe. He may obtain equal numbers from both parents or more from one or the other. Most likely the parent whose family has the greatest loading of schizophrenia provides the greatest number of genes. It is, of course, possible that anxiety or stress acting in some way on the biochemistry of the body can help trigger the process, but if this is a factor, it seems of little importance.

Biochemical Changes

The nerve cell or neuron is one of the main cells of the nervous system. It starts electrical impulses and transmits them to other neurons, and is essential to the working of the brain. It burns foodstuff to provide it with the energy it needs, and releases heat and waste chemicals. Neurons are surrounded by, and bathed in, body fluids. They control secretion of hormones and other chemicals about them.

The brain has an extraordinary need for energy. Just over two pounds of brain in a 150-pound man uses one quarter of the amount of energy used by the whole man at rest.

The point of connection—or bridge—between the neurons is called the synapse. Messages are carried across this bridge in an unusual way. When a neuron is stimulated, an impulse races down the nerve cell to the end of the nerve. There it releases a chemical messenger which may be acetylcholine, serotonin or noradrenaline. This chemical slowly moves across the bridge and when it arrives at the other end, stimulates the next nerve cell. Thus messages from our eyes, ears and other organs are carried from cell to cell.

The brain depends for its normal functioning upon a proper formation, release and removal of these chemicals. Too little or too much of any of the chemical messengers can prevent the brain from working properly. In addition to the enzymes which make them, therefore, there must be enzymes (protein substances) which destroy them when their work is done. The brain has both kinds of enzymes available to maintain the chemical messengers in proper quantities.

When poisons are formed in the brain, or penetrated into it from the blood, they can interfere with the work of these enzymes and prevent the removal of the messengers. The latter, therefore, continue to stimulate neurons when they should not, and can produce many abnormalities in brain operation, including convulsions. For example, many insect poisons block the action of the enzyme which destroys acetylcholine. This is why they are so poisonous for man if he should breathe them in or get them on his skin.

When anything happens to interfere with the way messages are normally transmitted across the synapse from one neuron to another, many other parts of the brain are thrown out of order. The disturbances which result can be seen when the electrical brain waves are measured by the electroencephalogram. This is what happens in schizophrenia.

Patients with schizophrenia have many abnormalities on their brain wave patterns. This has been established beyond doubt by the work of Professors Robert Heath, Stephen Sherwood, C. Shagass, L. A. Hurst, F. A. Gibbs, L. Goldstein and many others.

We believe that in schizophrenia, poisons made in the body interfere with the carrying of messages, and as a result those parts of the brain which keep the world around us steady, or, to use a technical term, maintain constancy of perception, are disturbed. We think these poisons include increased quantities of adrenochrome, adrenolutin, taraxein and other substances.

Although we shall, for simplicity's sake, write as if adrenochrome can only come from adrenaline, it is quite possible that other chemicals in the body might also be changed into adrenochrome. Professor Mark Altschule believes it might come from substances made in the body from the amino-acid, tyrosine. It is even possible adrenochrome-like chemicals can be made in the body from serotonin, but much more work is needed to settle this matter.

Adrenaline itself is very poisonous and too much of it can lead to serious changes. Physicians know this and rarely inject more than one milligram in one dose. There is enough stored in the body which, if released suddenly, would kill the subject. If it is secreted in the body in excessive quantities, it produces most of the symptoms of severe anxiety, panic, fear, and so on, increases blood pressure, causes headaches, and may cause haemorrhages in the body and brain.

Because adrenaline is so toxic, it must be removed as quickly as possible before it can do any damage. This is done naturally in the body where it is quickly changed into a large number of other compounds. Most of these are not dangerous or toxic, and in fact they may serve a useful role in the operation of the brain and body.

Recently it has been discovered that blood contains an enzyme called "adrenaline oxidase" which combines adrenaline with hydrogen peroxide to form new compounds. Adrenaline oxidase is an adaptive enzyme. In other words, the more adrenaline there is secreted into blood, the more enzyme is formed, presumably to protect the body from the toxic adrenaline.

Some of the adrenaline, however, is converted into another poisonous chemical, probably within the cells of the tissues and not outside them in the fluids which bathe them. This chemical, adrenochrome, has no effect on blood pressure and fortunately is very reactive, changing quickly in the body to less active chemicals. It is, however, poisonous to nerve cells and even trace quantities of pure adrenochrome, as Professor Ruth Geiger has shown, will kill them. It must, therefore, be removed as quickly as possible, and this can be done in two ways.

Protective or buffer substances in the body fluids quickly bind adrenochrome and keep it from coming in contact with the neuron. Adrenochrome can also be changed quickly into other, non-toxic chemicals. We are not certain we know all the substances which are needed to change adrenochrome into these non-toxic substances. This change requires enzymes, or catalysts. It is known to occur more easily when Vitamin C, the interesting amino-acid derivative, glutathione, and cysteine are present in sufficient amounts.

The non-toxic substance which is formed when adrenochrome is changed in this way is called 5,6,dihydroxy-N-methyl-indole (or leuco-adrenochrome). It has helped many subjects with its definite anti-tension properties. We consider the conversion of adrenochrome into leuco-adrenochrome a normal reaction in the body. We also believe there must be a balance between adrenaline and this substance. If there is a lot of adrenaline and not enough leuco-adrenochrome the subject will be anxious and tense. If there is enough leuco-adrenochrome, the balance is adequate and any anxiety in the person will be normal.

Leuco-adrenochrome is broken down further into a type of chemical called pyrolles, or built up into the brown or black pigments in the skin or in the brain.

But for reasons unknown, the adrenochrome in schizophrenia

is changed primarily into adrenolutin which is just as poison for animals in producing changes in behavior. As a result, schizophrenic patient has too much adrenochrome and much adrenolutin.

Physiologists and biochemists have studied adrenochrome since it was first identified in 1937, and a good deal is known about its actions in the body. Schizophrenic patients who have too much adrenochrome (and adrenolutin) will have certain biochemical abnormalities which are due to this poisonous substance.

The following changes are, therefore, most likely present in schizophrenics. The evidence is reported in our book, *The Chemical Basis of Clinical Psychiatry.* *

There will be a lowering of energy production in the brain. Foodstuff will be converted into energy less efficiently. This might account for the profound fatigue present in the majority of patients who have schizophrenia.

There is a chemical in the brain called gamma amino butyric acid (GABA) which is considered to be a regulator of transmission across the synapse. It prevents too many stimuli from jumping across the synapse. If too little is present, the brain will be too excitable and may even develop electrical storms which produce convulsions. GABA is made from the amino acid, glutamic acid, by the loss of one molecule of carbon dioxide. The enzyme which makes it is prevented from doing so by adrenochrome.

Thus, when adrenochrome is present, there will not be enough GABA and the brain, agitated by an over abundance of stimuli, will be too excitable or irritable. In fact, the majority of schizophrenic patients are irritable and have abnormal brain wave charges.

Adrenochrome also blocks the action of the enzyme which destroys acetylcholine. This is one of the messenger chemicals that crosses the synapse from the nerve cell to the neuron. There will then be too much acetylcholine in the synapse, and this will add to the irritability or excitability of the brain.

Schizophrenics have diabetes much less frequently than one would expect, and this can be due to the presence in their bodies

*The Chemical Basis of Clinical Psychiatry (Charles C. Thomas, Springfield, Illinois. 1960).

of adrenochrome and adrenolutin, which act the same way in the body as the compounds used to treat diabetes. Insulinase is the enzyme which destroys insulin and is too active in some forms of *diabetes mellitus.* These diabetic conditions are treatable by giving patients compounds which block the action of insulinase. Adrenochrome and adrenolutin act in the same way as these compounds and so often prevent diabetes from developing. However, it is possible for people who get diabetes first to develop schizophrenia later.

It had been observed some time ago that when schizophrenia comes on early in life, it prevents normal growth and development. The victims then tend to be slender, slight, and too narrow in the chest from front to back. There are also changes in each half of the body so that they develop what is called asymmetry (the shape of one half of the body does not conform to the shape of the other). If the disease comes on after physical growth is complete, no such malformation is possible.

Adrenochrome is a very powerful inhibitor of cell division and is known as a cell mitosis poison. In fact, this was one of the first properties of adrenochrome to be discovered long before we began to suspect it was related to schizophrenia. It should also interfere with all those processes in the body which depend upon the rapid growth of tissues. For example, when a tissue is injured it is normally repaid by a rapid growth of fibrous tissue. Tuberculosis lesions in the lung in normal people are walled in by this growth of fibrous tissue, and so do not spread through the lung.

But schizophrenic patients are less resistant to tuberculosis, probably because of too much adrenochrome in their bodies. Fortunately modern sanitation, better hospitals and antibiotic treatment have markedly reduced tuberculosis infection cases, and modern mental hospitals have tuberculosis in their schizophrenics nearly under normal control.

Other effects of reduced growth will appear in a slower rate of growth of hair, which we have observed in some patients, in a slower growth of nails, and in defective formation of sperms.

Adrenochrome also renders schizophrenic patients more prone to develop scurvy. Scurvy was once one of the most dreaded scourges of man, especially after a late winter when no fresh vegetables were available. It develops in the absence of Vitamin C, one of the essential chemicals found in foods.

Vitamin C is essential for normal body function and, since it cannot be made in the body, it must be taken in the food. Adrenochrome, however, combines with Vitamin C and so uses it up more quickly, leaving a deficiency in the schizophrenic.

Professor M. H. Briggs has shown that when scurvy is artifically induced in guinea pigs, they excrete certain unusual compounds in the urine. He has also shown that patients who have schizophrenia excrete the same substances.

The dark pigments in skin come from the amino-acid tyrosine, from dopamine and possibly from adrenochrome. Pigmented areas in the brain more likely come from adrenochrome. By contrast, albinos who have little or no color in the skin because they cannot form melanin from tyrosine, have normal melanin-like pigment in the brain. Albinos do not have any deficiency in the formation of adrenaline pigments.

Schizophrenics who have too much adrenochrome should, therefore, have darker skin than when they are not ill. Thus, we have found that elderly schizophrenic patients do not turn grey nearly as quickly as do other psychiatric patients. Lea has found that young patients with schizophrenia darken their hair color earlier than do subjects in the control group. The excess of dark pigment probably accounts for the extraordinary youthful appearance of many middle-aged and elderly patients.

The rare occurrence of allergic diseases or arthritis in schizophrenic patients is an observation which has been made frequently and had never been denied, but it is ignored by most psychiatrists. The reason for this favorable condition may be due to the presence of adrenochrome, which is an anti-histamine nearly as powerful as some of the weaker commercially made anti-histamines. Small quantities of adrenochrome constantly present in the body could protect schizophrenics against allergies more effectively than larger doses taken by non-schizophrenics a few times a day by mouth.

Schizophrenics also have a remarkable resistance to histamine. Histamine is a powerful substance found in small quantities in the body. When it is injected under the skin or into a vein, it produces a marked facial flush and a rapid drop in blood pressure. For this reason, only small quantities can be given without danger to the subject.

In 1952, early in our research program, one of our colleagues, Dr. John Lucy, found that chronic schizophrenic patients could tolerate remarkable quantities of histamine before the blood pressure went down. We were not trying to discover how much they could take. We were studying the effect of histamine injections as a treatment.

The procedure called for giving increased quantities of histamine until the blood pressure went down to a given degree. But when we began our studies with schizophrenia we found that so much histamine was needed to lower blood pressure, we quickly used up all our research supply. We asked a drug firm to make us solutions of histamine ten times as concentrated as before. This request was so unusual the firm was reluctant to do so unless we gave them a special release, since they had not previously known these large quantities could be given to subjects.

Schizophrenic patients are also more resistant to small quantities of histamine placed in the skin. Normally this produces a weal or a reddish raised area. But in schizophrenia the area of the weal is smaller and comes on more slowly.

The ability of schizophrenics to resist histamine is probably due to the presence of adrenochrome in increased concentrations. The greater supply of adrenochrome may also account for the remarkable resistance of schizophrenics to medical and surgical shock.

We will refer to only one more finding. Until recently serious studies were made of schizophrenics' brains, which were compared to the normal. Only the outer layers were studied, and although some changes were found in them, so many other factors could have been the cause that these findings are no longer taken seriously. In fact, the majority of psychiatrists now assume there are no changes in the brain in schizophrenia at all.

But very few studies have been made of the deeper areas of the brain which are particularly concerned with emotion. We believe no changes in the brain are found unless the disease has been present many years. But there is a good deal of evidence that, after ten years of illness, there are changes in the brain which lead to the enlargement of the brain ventricles. This is one of the important reasons for preventing early schizophrenia from becoming chronic schizophrenia by the best possible chemical treatment. For when neurons are destroyed, they can never be replaced, and when too many are gone, they set a permanent pattern of activity in the brain which may be as irreversible as the permanent weakening of cloth when too many fibres are removed from it.

There is one known way the body has of protecting its vital tissues against the poisonous chemical, adrenolutin, which comes from adrenochrome.

In normal men and women, the blood contains a protein called ceruloplasmin. It is a blue copper-containing substance which can change adrenaline to other substances, and which can also alter serotonin. One can easily measure, biochemically, how much is present in the blood. Ceruloplasmin has the remarkable property of being able to hold or bind adrenolutin so firmly it does not come off. If a small quantity of adrenolutin was released in the body, the ceruloplasmin would immediately soak or mop it up, and no harm could be done to the body.

During stress more adrenaline is secreted, and so it makes sense to suspect that a small quantity might then be converted into adrenochrome and adrenolutin. But during stress and physical disease there is also more ceruloplasmin in the blood, ready to mop up these harmful chemicals before they can do any damage, much as though the body has prepared itself to cope with such an eventuality.

Ceruloplasmin, because of its ability to remove adrenolutin, has been found to play an important role in the recovery of schizophrenics. It is made in the placenta, and during the last three months of pregnancy more is secreted from the placenta into the mother's blood. The mother is thereby protected against toxic substances like adrenolutin or histamine. On the other hand, after the baby is born, the amount of ceruloplasmin in the blood very quickly decreases and reaches normal levels in about two weeks.

This increased quantity of ceruloplasmin in pregnancy would be of great benefit in absorbing any abnormal quantities of adrenolutin present in the body. Once pregnancy is over, however, the woman is deprived of the extra ceruloplasmin, which means that the adrenolutin is free to exert its toxic effects. In fact, nearly two-thirds of all serious psychoses which occur after the baby is born, do come on within this short period after birth. Men also have ceruloplasmin in small quantities.

Professor Heath found that some schizophrenic patients had more ceruloplasmin than others and that these were the ones who more often recovered. This suggests they were able to recover because they had better biochemical defences against the disease, including the ability to make more ceruloplasmin. Dr. B. Melander has shown that ceruloplasmin injections will cure the majority of acute schizophrenics to whom it is given.

These early experiments have not been reproduced perhaps because as the ceruloplasmin preparations became more refined the active therapeutic principle was removed. It is not likely these results were due to a placebo reaction. These early positive experiments will remain a mystery.

Taraxein, Professor Heath's toxic protein, plays an important role in the formation of schizophrenia. Dr. Melander, on the basis of his research, suggested that taraxein might sensitize the brain to substances like adrenolutin. Over their evolutionary history, mammals have developed mechanisms for keeping most undesirable chemicals away from the brain. There is a barrier called the blood-brain barrier which keeps these toxic substances out. But Melander believes taraxein lowers the barrier and so substances like adrenolutin are able to penetrate into the brain more easily.

Both Melander and Heath have shown that, in animals, taraxein appears to increase the effect of even small quantities of adrenolutin. When animals are first given taraxein in small amounts, which do not produce changes in behavior and then given small quantities of adrenolutin, there is a very marked change in behavior. The presence of taraxein would make subjects peculiarly sensitive to quantities of adrenolution which might otherwise not be dangerous. Schizophrenic patients having both are, therefore, vulnerable for two main reasons.

We have also suggested that taraxein might act by increasing the conversion of adrenochrome into adrenolutin, or it might combine with ceruloplasmin and so prevent it from functioning as an absorber for adrenolutin. These are conjectures which may, or may not, be supported by data in years to come. Nevertheless, it is certain taraxein does play an important role in producing schizophrenia.

Psychological Changes

We think that there are three major changes in the psychological state in schizophrenia which can account for nearly all of the symptoms. These are: (1) changes in perception, (2) changes in thinking, and (3) fatigue. In every case, the important symptoms are those which change the person.

Changes in perception, thought, mood, and therefore in activity determine what happens to personality and to the patient.

Personality is the outcome of the combined effect of the customs and prevailing ideas where one lives, of family and of education. Everything which happens to a person will help shape him. Every individual as a result has his own unique personality. Any alteration due to schizophrenia will change what is there to something new. At the same time, the personality which the patient has acquired by the time his illness descends upon him, will determine how the primary changes of schizophrenia will affect him. Thus, schizophrenia is different in every one.

Many schizophrenics will have hallucinations, for example, but these will differ in content and each patient will react differently.

After the illness is over, the patient will regain to some degree his previous personality, but there will always remain some alterations since the schizophrenic illness produces a profound experience. Like any experience, it leaves its stamp forever. Experiences in wartime, or the horrors of concentration camp, have affected the personalities of many people permanently.

The changes left by schizophrenia are often thought to be expressions of the illness when, in fact, the person is well, but altered by the disease. The changes can be beneficial or injurious, and they may be permanent. In the same way, a profound LSD-25 experience may leave a permanent imprint.

Perceptual Changes

Some schizophrenics realize their normal powers of perception have gone awry, while others don't. Thus some may see the changes as being real, and some as unreal. If the changes are accepted as not being real, they may produce anxiety, doubt and a turning inward, but they will not alter character and personality as much as if they are assumed to be true.

If these strange experiences are frequent or persist a long time, they are likely to be accepted as real because man has always trusted his senses. It would be extremely doubtful if any one of us, who saw a man standing in front of him for a long time, would doubt there was someone.

Changes may come about in any of the senses. It is obvious that changes in some senses will not be as dangerous as changes in others. A perceptual change which interferes with a person's occupation will tend to be more harmful than those which attack other aspects of perception.

One of our patients, a stenographer, found that whenever she transcribed from one page to another, she could not keep her eyes on the line because it would jump to the line above or below. She tried to prevent this by placing a ruler under each line, but this did not help. She had other symptoms but this is the one which made it impossible for her to do her job and forced her into hospital.

In general, vision and sound are distance senses which chiefly determine one's relations to our fellow men. Smell, taste and touch are intimate senses and are used to control relations with lovers, close friends and relatives. Thus it is likely that sight and sound are going to produce hostile reactions more often. Schizophrenia is usually not diagnosed until vision and hearing are altered and the patient has responded with fear or anger, or in some other way which draws attention to him.

Any visual change will be reacted to in a common sense way. We mean this that anyone with imagination can place himself in a similar situation and predict fairly accurately what the expected reaction would be. We will merely list some with no elaboration.

CHANGES	RESULTS
People are watching	Suspicion, uncertainty (paranoid behavior)
Faces are distorted	Fear, suspicion
Faces are funny	Inappropriate giggling
Inability to distinguish faces	Confusion, suspicion
Colors too bright	Euphoria
Colors dull	Depression
Unable to judge distance	Fear, anxiety when driving
Hallucinations	Depends on kind

Subtle changes can be just as injurious as gross ones, although the subject may be unaware of them. For example, when two people are talking to one another they use a tone of voice just loud enough for clear transmission of words. But sound waves follow the inverse square law. When the distance between people is doubled, the voice must be raised four times for the same intensity of sound to be transmitted. The speaker must be able to judge how far he is before he can adjust his voice properly. This is not a conscious decision except with speaking on a public platform when the speaker knows he must make an effort to get his voice to the back of the hall.

Suppose, due to a defect in judging distance, the patient doesn't know how far away he is from the person to whom he is talking. Then he may speak too softly, thinking the other person is close, or too loudly, thinking the other person is too far. But the one to whom he is talking is unaware of this. What he notices is that he is being shouted at or whispered to, and this can easily result in difficulties in communication.

Some patients have a defect in estimating distance on the road. This makes driving an anxious business, and our patients are often reluctant or unable to drive. If the patient is a truck driver, he will lose his job. But it could be much worse if he had not been aware of something being wrong.

Some people respond quite appropriately oo their hallucinations. One young woman saw Christ, who told her she was destined to be his bride. She thereupon gave up her job, went home to her parents, and spent her days studying the Bible and telling her parents about the hallucinations. This led to her admission to hospital.

Patients often feel that both their eyes and ears may be playing tricks on them, especially as the illness comes on or as they begin to recover. Many schizophrenics have described their doubts that what they were seeing was real. One of these was Perceval, the son of a British Prime Minister in the 19th century, who became schizophrenic, recovered, and then wrote his own account of his illness in *Perceval's Narrative*.

Perceval expressed some anger and resentment toward his brother because, when he experienced hallucinations and asked his brother about them, the latter did not tell him they were hallucinations. For many months Perceval believed the voices he heard were real and prophetic. Later on in his illness, as he began to recover, he used several ingenious psychological experiments to help him decide whether they were real or not. For example, at the height of his illness, he was convinced that every prophecy made by his voices was true. But later he kept track of the prophecies and soon observed that most of the time they did not occur. He decided the voices were fallible, and later that they were not real. Judge Schreber also tested the reality of his hallucinations while in mental hospital, and found them unreliable at times.

AUDITORY CHANGES

Sounds may be too low or too intense. We have seen patients come to hospital because their hearing was too acute and they could hear people talking several rooms away. In our work with Dr. S. Fogel we found that when hearing was made too keen, our subjects became suspicious, angry, and extremely distractible. They developed hallucinations of hearing. They reacted to an extreme degree to any extraneous sounds coming from within the room or from outside, and it was difficult to engage them in conversation.

The ability to know where sound is coming from is most important during the formative years, particularly in infancy when eye and ear must be nicely coordinated. When infants cannot tell where their mother's voice comes from, they do not respond normally and may even seem to be deaf. There cannot be a normal communication between mother and child—mother smiling and talking to child, child smiling back and gurgling . . . for the child does not know the voice is coming from the mother, and it is difficult for them to establish an emotional bond between them.

Patients will, of course, respond to voices if these are believed to be real. The response will depend on what the voices say. We do not need to remind the reader that if the voices are accepted as true they will be responded to, argued with and acted upon. Many patients hear voices which are hallucinations, but to the patients these are real voices telling them what to do. Some of our patients were told not to eat and they began to starve even though they were very hungry. The worst kind of communication is one where voices order the listener not to take medication.

TASTE PERCEPTION

It has been known for many years that people's taste sensations differ. The same tea may have a different taste to everyone who drinks it. The ability to taste a compound called phenylthiocarbamide is inherited. To some people it tastes bitter and to others it is tasteless.

It is remarkable how often people will not believe that this difference in taste is possible. Tasters do not believe there are non-tasters, and non-tasters believe tasters are lying or are mentally sick. Husband and wife have been observed to have furious arguments over this. This is due to the nearly universal belief that every person senses the common world like every other person, and all things are seen, felt, taste, smelled the same way by all people.

It is also believed that, if there are changes in taste, this must be due to a clearly recognizable condition, such as having a cold, being tired, and so on. When, therefore, changes in taste sensation do come on in the absence of a cold or other such reason to blame it on, it is assumed to be due to a change in the food that is being eaten. Coffee may suddenly taste bitter, or something has been put in the meat to make it taste strange.

One of the most distressing things that can happen is for food to taste bitter, metallic or tainted, for this can easily lead to the belief it has been poisoned. Many patients will, as a result, refuse to eat, and will suffer malnutrition.

The poisoning delusion leads some people to prepare their own food in elaborate and peculiar ways, and has led some patients to take drastic action in self-defence against the alleged poisoner.

Other taste changes may puzzle and bewilder, but they need not lead to any great inconvenience unless, of course, the patient is a taster whose livelihood depends upon the sense of taste. Though, if this happens to a wife, who is usually the cook cn the family, it might account for some peculiar taste in the food of which she would be unaware, but which might lead to bitter arguments with the rest of the family.

SMELL PERCEPTION

Normal human beings are as loath to accept the fact that the same things smell differently to everyone as they are to believe they taste differently. Yet it is well known that some people find a perfume most attractive when others will consider the same perfume to be vile. Generally, children are better smellers than adults. There are cases reported of children who were able to identify the owners of clothes by the unique odor, even after the clothes had been cleaned.

Many physicians can diagnose certain diseases by the odor. We can smell schizophrenia when it is present in some subjects, while other physicians cannot. The smell of schizophrenia is a peculiar, aromatic slightly musty odor. Many schizophrenics can smell their own sick odor and find it very troublesome. One of our female patients diagnosed the condition in three out of her seven children by this odor. As they recovered, the odor vanished.

Changes in smell perception can result in a variety of bizarre delusions. Several patients have smelled strange odors and assumed they were being gassed. Others have assumed food was poisoned, because of the smell, and refused to eat it. This recalls the work of Professor Kurt Richter with rats. When given poisoned food they had a choice of eating or of starving. Instead, they became catatonic.

One patient complained someone was pulling his seminal fluid from him since he could smell it all over himself. We have already mentioned another of our patients who made desperate attempts to deodorize his barn because his sense of smell had become too keen. One patient kept smelling dust and insisted on a thorough housecleaning every day. When her family objected she became violently angry. A whole family can be subjected to elaborate bathing and washing rituals by a sick member.

TOUCH PERCEPTION

This rarely bring patients into hospital. We can recall one whose chief complaint was a feeling that worms were crawling under his skin. Touch misperceptions are probably responsible for patients feeling that they are being afflicted by electricity, rays, and mysterious influences from cosmic forces. Closely allied to touch misperception are alterations in the sensing of heat and cold.

It is possible alterations in the sensations of touch in the genital areas lead to the delusions some patients have that someone is tampering with their sexual organs. Usually libido (sex urge) is decreased, perhaps because of the decrease in the sensibility to touch of the genitals.

TIME PERCEPTION

Misperceptions of time are very common in schizophrenic patients. This is especially true of patients who have been treated in mental hospitals for long periods of time. It is difficult to decide whether this is due to the disease or whether it is due to the prolonged stay in hospital. The normal aids for facilitating time perception, such as clocks, calendars, newspapers and visitors, are strikingly absent in mental hospitals. But even when these are present, there still remains a good deal of time misperception.

The effect of being unable to judge the passing of time is easily demonstrated by hypnotic techniques, which we described in Chapter III.

CHANGES IN THOUGHT

Our perception affects our thoughts. We depend on our senses to help us formulate ideas and adapt to our surroundings. Those of us who perceive normally can change our ideas more readily than those who do not. For it is when our surrounding world is stable that we are free to think.

A child learning to walk, for example, is so preoccupied with his task he can do little else at the moment. But once he can walk easily he can consider other matters. Similarly, some schizophrenics are so distracted by the continual assault of sounds when hearing is magnified, or by bright colors or details in objects when colors are intensified, that they cannot keep their minds on other matters.

The chief change in schizophrenia, therefore, seems to be an increasing inability to change one's point of view. Patients seem less able than normal people to examine a question from various points of view and to judge whether their perceptional world is real or not. But we may be unfair about this. A normal person who sees people watching him may be just as rigid in believing this to be true as any paranoid schizophrenic.

A delusional system often arises from perceptual changes and these in turn are due to faulty interpretation of signals by the brain. For example, if a patient hears a radio announcer saying obscene things about him, he is likely to believe the radio station is against him and act accordingly. These changes place the sick person at a great disadvantage in his dealings with his fellow men.

Mood

Everyone is sad, blue or depressed now and then. Nearly everyone feels depressed when he is ill, indisposed or finds himself in difficult situations. The usual early symptom of schizophrenia is depression because life becomes uncertain, frustrating, confused and difficult. Only later, as the disease advances, does depression lift, to be followed by the even more frightening inability to feel any emotion.

It is a common error to diagnose schizophrenia in its early phases as depression. Professor Nolen D. C. Lewis many years ago found that nearly half of a large group of depressed patients treated at the New York Neuropsychiatric Institute were later rediagnosed as schizophrenic.

Fatigue

One of the most common changes in schizophrenia is fatigue. Very often it is the first symptom to appear. It comes on slowly and insidiously and is very disabling. It becomes difficult to perform one's job and this produces great anxiety. Eventually fatigue may become so great that the patient is immobilized by it. Others, not realizing how ill he is, find this difficult to understand and patients, as a result, are often accused of being lazy and indifferent. The latter naturally resent this, and so further misunderstanding are resentment is generated.

One of our male patients, aged 26, recalled recently the great difficulty he had had because of fatigue. He had been ill many years, with several admissions to a mental hospital. He suffered an acute episode about two years ago, and was admitted for a day as an emergency. He was started on nicotinic acid which he has taken regularly since. The past few months he has been taking a special re-education course in order to complete secondary school.

Recently he remarked that he clearly recalled the excessive fatigue he first felt when he was eight years old. This feeling remained with him from then until after he had taken the vitamin for about one year. During those seventeen intervening years he was chronically fatigued and considered to be lazy, stupid and indifferent. With some bitterness he recounted the great difficulty he had had in school, and said that he had always considered himself to be stupid. But now he found he was able to grasp the course of studies with little difficulty, and realized he was not stupid at all, but had had trouble learning because he had been ill.

Social Factors

The social consequences of schizophrenia follow naturally from the perceptual and other disturbances which accompany the illness. Yet as far as we know, they have never been linked together in an understandable way.

Perhaps by examining some of the simplest interactions between two people, we can become aware of a few of the many problems which assail not only the sick person, but the well with whom he comes in contact.

As Professor Edward T. Hall has shown, the presence of a person who does nothing and says nothing will alter the behavior of someone who has previously been alone.

Let us suppose, then, that two people are walking towards each other. At first they are too far away for recognition to be possible. But then they get closer, and it might seem that up to this point nothing much could possibly go wrong. Yet we know from the work of our old friends, Professors Sommer and T. Weckowicz, that much could, and very often, does go wrong.

As people walk toward us, we see them getting closer. But they also get bigger and bigger. We learn to interpret this enlarging of the image on the eye retina as meaning the individual is getting closer, although it might equally well mean that the object from which the light was being reflected was getting larger.

This is a subtle distinction which schizophrenic patients are sometimes unable to make, and many of them have reported the eerie and frightening experience of a tiny dwarf becoming a huge and menacing giant as it looms forward.

In normal people, by some complex and not yet understood mechanism of the brain, the approaching figure remains roughly the same size, but for many schizophrenics, we now know, this reassuring mechanism goes wrong.

A very common problem these patients face, for instance, occurs when they are driving on the highway and oncoming cars seem to rush by too quickly. In addition, they are uncertain of their position in their own car lane, and many feel they are too close to the center line or too close to the edge of the road. For this reason, it is not unusual for patients who are developing schizophrenia to stop driving many months before they seek help. Others, however, continue to drive, and we suspect the accident rate for schizophrenics is rather high.

We know one patient who was an excellent pilot of small planes and made a living dusting crops. He was normal as long as he took nicotinic acid regularly. For unknown reasons, he stopped taking the medication, and a few months later his symptoms began to reappear. While motoring back to Saskatoon for help he drove his car into a concrete pier alongside the road and was killed.

A second patient was a physician who became schizophrenic. He also died in a similar car accident. Finally we have recently come upon a schizophrenic patient who has a long record of automobile accidents. He might well be called accident prone.

We have produced similar changes in normal subjects by giving them adrenochrome. One subject was a well known and a very good research psychiatrist. He was given 10 mg. of adrenochrome which he dissolved under his tongue. A couple of hours later as we were driving him away in a car he was suddenly surprised to see trees exploding in his field of vision as we drove alongside them.

What the sick person does about this strange experience must depend on his previous life's experiences. He may simply be interested, observe it and learn how to live with it. His stoic calm is perhaps more frequent than we suppose. One of us (A.H.) took sublingual (under the tongue) adrenochrome. For two days after that he found that objects seemed to be either a little larger or a little smaller. This was interesting rather than disturbing, but of course there was a logical explanation.

A patient seeing the same things may equally well become panic stricken, freeze with fear, run away or lash out with his fists. When he sees someone coming toward him as being frighteningly large, whatever he does is likely to surprise and even distress the other person.

If the latter is genial and expansive, he may be holding out a hand in welcome, but the sick one will see an enlarged and quickly growing hand coming at him in an uncanny or menacing way. As fear and terror grows, this hand could lose all connection with his friend's body, and as it seemingly pounces on him it might turn into a huge disembodied talon clawing forward.

A schizophrenic person can easily confuse his wishes and hopes about a relationship which might develop in the future with one that actually exists in the present. Actions taken on the basis of these unrealistic hopes may well confuse and dismay the other person. The schizophrenic would then feel that he had been brutally and inexplicably rebuffed by someone whom he had deeply trusted.

Schizophrenic patients sometimes fail to recognize those who are familiar to them. This is not surprising if one considers how extraordinary it is that we can pick out people we know, from hundreds or even thousands of people who are roughly the same size and shape. Orientals often complain that all Occidentals look alike, and *vice versa*. This suggests that we commonly use rather small clues to distinguish one face from another.

The schizophrenic who doesn't recognize his friend will suppose that he is being addressed in a familiar way by a stranger, and may refuse to acknowledge his greeting, turn away, suggest that he has made a mistake, or respond in a reserved or perfunctory manner. This may hurt the friend's feelings enough for the sick person to lose contact with someone who, if he had understood what was happening, would have made allowances for such behavior in the very same way that one excuses short-sightedness or deafness.

It may happen that the sick person mistakes a total stranger for a relative, friend or an enemy, often due to some real resemblance. Anyone who has waited those long minutes which seem like hours for a girl friend at some assigned spot knows how frequently girls, as seen in the distance, can resemble each other in size. As the figure comes closer, hopes rise only to be dispelled when you are about to greet the wrong one.

Expectations are great deceivers. The schizophrenic person can easily mistake a similarity for an identity and refuse to believe that a total stranger is not a relative or a close friend. He will then address the stranger in an unexpectedly warm and friendly way. This is often reciprocated, for most of us are usually delighted with such spontaneous friendliness. This, however, only confirms the sick person's belief, and disillusionment follows sooner or later, making him timid and uncertain about initiating such relationships in the future. He may easily come to believe that doubles of his relatives and friends are being kept near him to annoy or spy upon him. Schizophrenic patients need constant warmth and encouragement and they respond to this slowly but positively. Unluckily they are easily put off by what they construe to be rejection, and take it very much to heart.

Time perception plays a big part in social relationships. Speech which is either too fast or too slow, becomes unintelligible.

Speech depends upon loudness, pitch, a variety of emphasis and inflection, all of which are influenced by timing and which can greatly alter the meaning of what is spoken. The simplest phrase can be said in many different ways with many different meanings. A skilled actor can make a sentence like "To be or not to be? That is the question", carry all kinds of unexpected possibilities.

But timing affects much simpler matters than speech—the handshake, for instance. Few of us know exactly how long a handshake ought to take. Most of us, however, do know when a handshake takes too short or too long a time. A person who drops one's hand without clasping it, or holds on to it indefinitely, gives one a sense of discomfort and uneasiness which is quite hard to put into words. Try it on an old friend and see what he makes of it, but be sure to explain what you have done afterwards.

Yet this ability to shake hands at the "right" speed is something which we learn during childhood from those around us, and which must be closely connected with our time sense and with an awareness that the person whose hand we are shaking feels that the ceremony is completed.

Again, just how close should one stand to another person? Professor Hall, in his brilliant series of studies, has shown that this differs greatly from country to country. Arabs, South Americans and Russians like to be close to a person with whom they are talking. North Americans and British prefer being further away and are literally stand-offish. Different peoples have different ideas about what these distances should be, but one usually learns the distances which one's neighbors, friends and relatives prefer, and most of us maintain them.

The schizophrenic person often loses his ability to judge the volume of his envelope of space around others and around himself. He either comes too close and and seems intrusive, or stands too far away and appears unfriendly. The consequence of either of these actions can be graver than one might expect. If someone intrudes on our personal space we tend to move away involuntarily, and if they keep coming towards us we become tense and anxious. The sick person may easily interpret this to mean a distaste for him personally, and either withdraw hurt and mortified, or become quarrelsome to revenge himself for the slight.

If it is the schizophrenic whose need for space around him has been increased, he may become afraid and angry at what seems to him to be an aggressive and unjustified intrusion upon his very being. Unless one knows what may be wrong, such behavior seems inexplicable, and indeed, it usually is, for nearly all of us take these everyday matters for granted because they are outside our awareness.

It is for this reason that we are so much obliged to Professors Hall, Sommer and Weckowicz, whose painstaking researches have focussed attention here.

These, then, are simple and straightforward examples of the way in which schizophrenia affects everyday life situations.

Let us look at something a little more complicated. In many, perhaps most situations involving two or more people, one is seen as being older, wiser, richer, more powerful, more important or higher-ranking than the others. This is known as a status relationship, and similar relationships occur among many gregarious animals and birds.

Examples among humans are employer and employee, teacher and pupil, mother and daughter, bishop and curate, officer and soldier, older brother and younger brother. The person of higher status is expected to behave in ways that show he is aware of his higher station, and the lower-status person to acquiesce with good grace. Most of us learn to accept a higher or lower status in a variety of rapidly altering situations. Indeed, in everyday life everyone of us has to be a quick-change artist in these matters.

We are parents one moment, and could be children the next; pupil in one situation, teacher in another; telling people what to do in the morning, and having our licenses scrutinized by the police in the afternoon. However, we can only succeed in such changes if we can perceive both ourselves and other people accurately. If we cannot do this, we are likely to behave strangely and make those with whom we are trying to interact, behave less normally too. A lower-status person is as uncomfortable with a higher-status person who behaves in a manner below his station as if the reverse occurred. A general who behaves towards a colonel as if the colonel were his superior would make the latter unhappy.

Schizophrenics can and do make both kinds of mistakes due to their misperceptions, and this leads to endless trouble. The tension and uncertainty is compounded because people are seldom aware of what is happening, and can take no adequate

counter-measures. Consequently, social relations become erod-
ed or may break down completely.   Due to his perceptual
difficulties and his lack of energy, the schizophrenic person
cannot respond to his fellows either as quickly or as consistently
as normals can. Unless healthy people know what is wrong, and
are taught how to help him and make allowances for his
deficiencies, he will probably drift, and be driven further and
further out of touch.

These are a few social difficulties arising in schizophrenia
which we have discussed sketchily. A systematic description of
what can happen lies outside the scope of this book and would
range beyond the boundaries of out still very limited knowledge.
There is a rich harvest of information, but the reapers are still far
too few.

Description of Schizophrenia Coming On in Various Periods of Life

DURING CHILDHOOD

Childhood is the period in life when schizophrenia can do the
most harm. The earlier the onset, the graver the consequences,
unless the illness disappears spontaneously or as a result of early
treatment.

The illness will have the most damaging effects if it comes on
either before or shortly after speech has fully developed. One of
the serious effects of the disease at this time is that vocalization
seems to stop. Normally, babies babble, and when from the
variety of gurglings and bleating, they produce one that seems to
make sense to mother (or father) there is an appropriate
response. The word "ma," for example, is responded to by
parents with great enthusiasm. This occurs until "ma" becomes
firmly attached to a person, mother. Thus words are learned so
gradually that we hardly realize what is happening, until the child
grasps the uses and symbolic meaning of words.

But if a child never babbles or vocalizes, there would be
nothing for parents to respond to, and so language could not
develop. Schizophrenic babies are unusually quiet, or make
single monotonous sounds to which parents cannot respond, and
we think this is why they cannot learn to speak. If it were possible

to stimulate babbling, perhaps they could learn to speak in the usual way. Young children who have learned a few words seem unable to learn more and often forget the ones they have already learned. It seems, therefore, that schizophrenia at this stage prevents the further learning of new words.

If the disease vanishes, the degree to which speech will recover depends upon the duration of the illness. There is a critical period of several years when speech is learned. If it is not learned within this period, it will not be learned at all, or at best it will be imperfect and rudimentary unless a major and sustained remedial effort is made by competent teachers.

Schizophrenic children seem to have many of their senses altered. They may have trouble recognizing people and, therefore, they do not learn to respond appropriately to their parents, who are understandably puzzled and disappointed. If hearing is affected, they may be unable to localize sources of sound and may, therefore, pay no attention to sounds. If the sounds ignored include those of mother calling, this can be very disruptive of the normal development of the mother-child relationship.

These children may have sufficient perceptual abnormalities that they will be unable to learn and will most likely be labelled mentally retarded. When this happens they are forced into the mold devised by society which keeps them segregated, in special schools, ill because it is assumed they have a condition which cannot be cured, and retarded because once labelled in this way it is very difficult to become unlabelled.

If the illness comes on after speech has developed, these children may stop speaking, but there is a better chance that speech will be re-established if the disease is properly treated. These years before puberty are crucial ones in human development, and a year lost here may be very difficult to regain. But the closer to adolescence the illness comes, the better the prognosis will be. Growth will be more affected at this time, of course, than after puberty. These children are often dark, slender, and narrow from front to back.

It is easy to find fault with parents at this period. There is no doubt that the mother-child relationship is disturbed. The prime reason is that the junior partner, due to illness, does not behave the way a normal child does. The mother, therefore, is left unrewarded for all the love, attention and care given to her child, and becomes irritable, frustrated and worried. This does not help her in her care for a very sick child.

If mother herself, which occasionally happens, is somewhat disposed to schizophrenia, it might be even more difficult for her to react appropriately. The system of rewards and punishment which worked with her normal children no longer applies and an impossible situation is created. Her problem is not made easier by those psychiatrists, psychologists, social workers and others who have, on slender evidence, decided that mother has made her child ill.

The only hope for these children is early identification of the illness. Just as special diets may be too late after one month in phenyl pyruvic oligophrenia (a form of retardation caused by lack of a protein enzyme) so with schizophrenic children. They must be recognized as early as possible by skilled psychiatrists, who will use the mauve factor urine test if necessary to help them.

Between 1965 and 1972 there has been an expansion of megavitamin therapy for many children who are not schizophrenic but who have various learning and behavioral problems. This newer work is best shown by reprinting portions of papers which appeared in *Schizophrenia*, published by the American Schizophrenia Association, by Hoffer.

Vitamin B-3 Dependent Child

A. Hoffer, M.D., Ph.D., F.A.P.A.

It is difficult to work with children. Diagnosis of disturbed children is in a very chaotic state, there being close to 50 different diagnostic terms for hyperactive or hyperkinetic children. They range from perceptually disturbed children, to minimal brain disorders, hyperkinetic disorders, schizophrenia and autistic children.

It occurred to me four years ago that we might be able to classify these disturbed children by their response to megadoses of vitamin B-3. Is there a syndrome that could be labelled "the vitamin B-3 responsive syndrome." This could be done by giving a fairly large number of disturbed and sick children ample quantities of vitamin B-3. Children who became well would then be examined for some constant features which could become an indication for using vitamin B-3. In principle it is the same as labelling every person who recovers on vitamin doses of B-3 as having suffered from pellagra or subclinical pellagra.

To examine this question, I began a single blind placebo controlled study three and one half years ago on children under age 13 who were referred to me because of disturbed and disturbing behavior. Many had been treated by various psychiatrists before this. This study will soon be completed, but certain conclusions are now evident.

Design

All seriously disturbed children referred to me by family physicians were carefully examined in my office and later by a colleague, Dr. B. O'Regan. They were then placed upon nicotinamide or, rarely, on nicotinic acid if there was no response to nicotinamide. The dose was increased from 1 to 6 gm. per day. They were also given ascorbic acid, 3 gm. per day and rarely very small doses of tranquilizers or antidepressants. They were then seen every three months to evaluate their progress. At no time were they given or were their parents given any dynamic psychotherapy.

As soon as the the child recovered, whether it took three months or two years, he was taken off nicotinamide and given the same dose of equivalent placebo tablets. The ascorbic acid and other chemotherapy was not altered. The child was not aware of any change in medication. The mother was—as I consider it medically unethical for me to use any more double blind experiments with vitamin B-3.

As long as the child remained well he was kept on placebo. But as soon as the parents were convinced that the child had regressed to a substantial level, they stopped the placebo and started him back on the nicotinamide.

After three years I made a final evaluation of each child taking into account his performance in school, his relation to his family and the presence of any symptoms. They were also re-evaluated by Dr. O'Regan.

Each child was given a diagnosis but irrespective of this, they were placed into the research group.

Results

Of the 38 children entering the study six were terminated before they had completed their three years.

Of these, one, a mongoloid child whose father is a recovered schizophrenic did not respond after six months and there seemed then no point in carrying on with him.

A second child was making excellent improvement but would not keep her appointments. Her parents seemed quite disinterested and she was dropped from the study.

A third child would not take his medication. Whenever he was forced to take his vitamin he would begin to recover but the battle between him and his parents was too difficult and eventually he was sent to a home for disturbed children.

The remaining three children were the products of a schizophrenic, alcoholic father who killed himself, leaving a severely schizophrenic widow. It was impossible for her to ensure her children's cooperation, nor was she herself able to cooperate.

Twenty-four children went through the treatment-placebo-treatment cycle. In each cases he or she recovered on treatment, relapsed on placebo within one month, and recovered again on vitamin B-3. In many cases, recovery was slower after a placebo-induced relapse.

The remaining eight are still in the first phase of the study, are well or nearly well and will this year go onto placebo.

Thus, of 33 children who took medication as directed, only one was a failure.

I should emphasize that by "well" or "recovered," I mean they are free of symptoms and signs, are performing well in school, getting on well with their families and with the community. Some are now in their early teens and members of Schizophrenics Anonymous.

Twenty-seven families were included in this study. In 13 families, neither father or mother were ill. Of their 47 children, 16 were included in the group, i.e., 34% of their children were ill. Since they were target families with at least one sick child, this is close to what one would expect, assuming an average family size of around three.

In nine families one parent had been ill and had recovered from a vitamin B-3 responsive illness, usually schizophrenia.

Six had sick fathers and three had sick mothers. Out of 29 children, 13 or about 45% were ill.

In five families both parents had schizophrenia. From 22 children, 18 or 82% were ill.

Discussion

Most of the children who were given the medication regularly recovered but a few parents were too ill or too indifferent to cooperate and their children's recovery was too interrupted by failure to maintain medication. In other words, most of the children are vitamin B-3 responsive.

The main variable was vitamin B-3 for when this was replaced by placebo all children had relapsed within 30 days. There was no change in ascorbic acid, in other medication or in nutrition.

In every case good nutrition was emphasized.

When vitamin B-3 was restarted, the children recovered again, although in many cases, more slowly.

Diagnosis of these children was as varied as with any group of disturbed children. The only thing in common was that they were ill, very disturbed and most were hyperactive. Diagnosis was no indicator of reponse.

Therefore, I must conclude that the condition which I term a vitamin B-3 dependent disease can manifest itself in a variety of forms. I consider it a vitamin B-3 dependent disease because they require 3 to 12 gm. per day of vitamin B-3 and because good diet alone has absolutely no effect upon them. My data shows that vitamin B-3 dependency is inherited. In more than 100 families that I have examined in the past 10 years, I find that if one parent is vitamin B-3 dependent, one quarter of the children also will be. If both parents are vitamin B-3 dependent, one will expect more than ¾ of the children also to be vitamin B-3 dependent.

There has so far been no generation gap. One can trace this from one generation to another. I have now in my care five patients including one mother, three of her nine children and one hyperkinetic grandchild, son of one of the three. The grandfather was a paranoid, depressed personality. Of his 10 children three including the mother of the nine were mentally ill with schizophrenia or retardation.

Another example comes from this controlled study and covers two generations. Peter and Mary are patients in this study.

Peter, 9 years old, was the first member of a vitamin B-3 dependent family who was referred to me for treatment. For over a month he had markedly changed from a happy, too quiet, obedient boy to one who was hostile, irritable and fearful. He was terribly worried he might give way to his murderous impulses against his parents or against himself. Thus, he was afraid to take a bath because he was afraid that he might drown himself. These fears had been present over one year but not at the same intensity. Peter described his life as a nightmare of visions, perceptual illusions and fears.

He was started on nicotinamide 1½ gm. per day, ascorbic acid 1½ gm. per day, and continued on Thorazine 50 mg. at bedtime.

After one month he was slightly better. After the third month he was even better. He reported hearing voices and a choir of voices singing church songs. His performance in school had improved substantially. He reported that rubbing his ears no longer masked out the voices the way it used to and he described a vision he had seen before starting on megavitamin therapy. He saw Christ sitting on a chair.

After 7 months he was normal. He was started on placebo while continuing with ascorbic acid and Thorazine. After two weeks he began to relapse and his behavior began to revert to his pre-treatment condition. He could no longer sleep, nightmares came back, objects seemed far away and he became fearful and disobedient. There was no doubt he had relapsed.

After one month of placebo he was placed back on nicotinamide and Thorazine was discontinued. Within a month he was well. When seen after three years I found him normal as did my colleague who had examined him earlier. He reported that Peter was "a normal 12-year-old boy."

Peter's HOD scores were:

1968	Total	Perceptual	Paranoid	Depression
January	76	18	2	11
April	56	14	3	8
July	36	9	4	3
October	13	1	1	2

Peter's sister, Mary, age 7, was next referred. She was considered retarded. She had started to walk late and had learned to speak slowly. For two years she was a placid, quiet baby. Then she became disturbed; suffered many temper tantrums. In 1963 she was severely retarded but in 1961 she was classed as dull normal. She went to kindergarten but was too disturbing to the class and she was sent to a class for the retarded. She had not responded to tranquilizers.

When I saw her, I did not consider her retarded as she was very alert, perceptive, but was typically hyperactive. She was noisy, irritable, short-tempered. She had a marked epicanthal fold which gave her a mongoloid appearance. She was started on nicotinamide and ascorbic acid, the dose increasing to 4½ gm. per day of vitamin B-3. She was also Thorazine and 200 mg. per day of Pyridoxine.

After six months there had been no improvement and the parents, in discouragement, stopped all medication. For one year she remained the same, but late in 1969 she began to hear voices and TV in her head. She was again started on nicotinamide 3 gm. per day, ascorbic acid 3 gm. per day, glutamic acid 2 gm. per day and Pyridoxine 100 mg. per day.

Improvement was very slight. In July, 1970 she became violently psychotic. She heard voices telling her to kill, she was in a constant panic and terribly fearful. It appeared she would have to be treated in an institution.

As a last resort she was started on nicotinic acid 12 gms. per day, ascorbic acid 3 gms. per day and, as a sedative, Dilantin 150 mg. per day. For the next month this family lived through a nightmare in which they had to give Mary 24-hour nursing care. Then she began to improve slowly.

When seen on March 5, 1971 she had shown dramatic improvement. She was relaxed, at ease no longer fearful, able to sleep alone, and getting on much better in school. It was very clear she was an intelligent girl slowly recovering from a very severe psychosis. If she maintains her present rate of improvement, she will be well by the end of 1971.

Peter's and Mary's father was referred next. He had been under psychiatric treatment for depression for two years. These episodes of depression had troubled him all his life. Medication had levelled out his mood to a chronic state of depression. He had read *How to Live With Schizophrenia* and concluded that he too suffered from schizophrenia.

When examined he was not very ill but he described having seen visions and other perceptual changes. He had also been paranoid in the past but his main complaint was depression and fatigue. As he was obese I ran the five-hour glucose tolerance test and found he had relative hypoglycemia. After six months of orthomolecular treatment he was well. (His father had been very irritable and suspicious for 10 years before he died at age 65.)

His HOD scores were:

1968	Total	Perceptual	Paranoid	Depression
January 16	27	5	0	6
April 2	15	3	0	4

The next family illustrates another two-generation transmission of vitamin B-3 dependency. Mr. J. D., born in 1933, was seen in 1967 because of severe marital disharmony. Their marriage was normal until their first baby died in 1957. Gradually the marriage deteriorated and was especially bad for the past five years. He had concluded that he and his wife must separate because he had no feeling toward her whatever and was sexually disinterested and impotent.

When examined he was very suspicious but admitted peculiar perceptual changes, complained that his memory was bad and was very depressed. He denied any paranoid ideas but these were reported to me by his wife. He also had a severe form of relative hypoglycemia.

He was started on vitamin B-3, 3 to 6 gm. per day, ascorbic acid 3 gm. per day, Elavil for one month and in three months was normal.

His HOD scores were down substantially:

	Total	Perceptual	Paranoid	Depression
Nov. 30, 1967	47	7	1	12
Dec. 14, 1967	62	14	3	6
Jan. 19, 1968	23	3	0	0

Early in January, 1968 the second child, a girl age 8, was brought in because her performance in school was so erratic, because of her violent temper, and because of a reading problem. Words moved on the page, faces pulsated, she saw vivid hallucinations, heard voices, and complained of being tired.

She was started on nicotinamide and ascorbic acid, 1 gm. of each per day. By May, 1968 she was normal. She was started on placebo to replace the nicotinamide. She deteriorated to her pre-treatment level within four weeks.

She was started again on nicotinamide but responded very slowly. The dose of nicotinamide was increased to 4 gm. per day by February, 1969. However, by October, 1970 she was well again and the dose was reduced to 2 gm. per day. At the end of the three years she was still normal.

There is a well-known vitamin deficiency disease which is an excellent model. Unfortunately psychiatrists are no longer familiar with the clinical manifestations of pellagra. When the older literature is examined, it is clear that the best model of schizophrenia is pellagra. It is so good that for many years psychiatrists in mental hospitals could not distinguish between them. The only certain diagnostic test was the therapeutic one, once crystalline vitamin B-3 became available. if the psychotic patient recovered in a matter of days on 1 gm. per day or less he was labelled pellagrin. If he did not he was retained in the diagnostic group "schizophrenia."

Both diseases are characterized by changes in perception, in thought and mood. The major difference has been in skin pigmentation. Pellagrins usually suffered symmetrical brown pigmentary changes while this was less common in schizophrenics. It is likely, however, this was an artifact resulting from the way the patients were cared for. Schizophrenics generally were locked up in mental hospitals and were not exposed to the sun, whereas pellagrins came in from the community and either recovered fairly quickly or died.

What is not as well known is that long before pellagrins became psychotic they suffered from tension, depression, personality problems, fatigue and every other change commonly seen in neurosis, psychopathies, depressions, etc. In other words, mild forms of pellagra modelled non-psychotic forms of pellagra and severe forms the psychotic varieties.

R. G. Green has treated a large number of disturbed children with nicotinamide. From the dramatic responses he has concluded they suffered from subclinical pellagra. His examination of the literature led him to the same conclusion as mine.

There is one major difference between pellagra and schizophrenia. It is entirely quantitative. Pellagrins require vitamin doses and schizophrenics require megavitamin doses. But even this distinction is not absolute. Chronic pellagrins, who should be compared with chronic schizophrenics, also require mega-doses for long periods of time.

There is thus a quantitative continum from pellagrins who fail to ingest vitamin doses of vitamin B-3, say 50 mg. per day or less, to chronic pellagrins who require up to 1 gm. per day, to acute schizophrenics whose needs are 3 to 6 gm. per day to chronic cases who will require 6 to 30 gm.

The group who require 50 mg. per day or less will develop pellagra if their diet is deficient. The group requiring over 1 gm. per day will develop schizophrenia since no modern diet will provide this amount of vitamin B-3. What I do not know is how much vitamin B-3 per day given to this latter group will prevent them from developing schizophrenia. To be on the safe side I recommend 1 gm. per day for children of parents who are vitamin B-3 dependent. One could study this very easily by placing a large number of children from schizophrenic parents on various doses to see how much is required to prevent anyone from becoming ill.

Conclusion

In my opinion based upon this study which I will report in detail later on, upon hundreds of other cases, my own and those reported by Cott and Hawkins, there is a syndrome in children arising from a vitamin B-3 dependency.

This syndrome is characterized by:

(1) Hyperactivity.
(2) Deteriorating performance in school.
(3) Perceptual changes.
(4) Inability to acquire or maintain social relationships.

Any child showing three or more of these features should be given a trial with the orthomolecular approach. In each case there should be a titering of dose until the child is exposed to the optimum dose. Once the child is recovered, it can be slowly reduced to a maintenance dose.

I do not know how long they will require vitamin B-3 but I suggest it not be discontinued until they have achieved their final physical growth. One schizophrenic girl has been taking vitamin B-3 for 17 years but will need it for the rest of her life. Another man stopped his vitamin at age 16 and is still well two years later.

A Vitamin B-3 Dependent Family

A. Hoffer, M.D., Ph.D.

Clinical Observations
Mr. E. S.

In 1954, Mr. E. S. began to suffer repeated episodes or "spells" of a peculiar type which he could not describe. He was admitted to University Hospital for treatment from February 26 to April 10, 1958, where a thorough investigation failed to yield any reason for his complaints. These peculiar episodes tended to come when Mr. E. S. was amongst people at times when he was very anxious. He described them as a feeling of boiling up inside during which he was weak and faint. His eyes went haywire and he felt a surge of something flash through his head. (Later he discovered these were transient mini-psychotomimetic experiences.)

The psychiatrist described this patient as an aggressive, very successful, very intelligent business man who had no interest in anything but his business. He was diagnosed as an obsessive compulsive neurosis with a paranoid personality.

Fortunately for Mr. E. S. he also had hypercholesterolemia (345 mg. per 100 ml. of blood) and several troublesome xanthomatoma on his eyelids. At a teaching conference the majority of physicians present agreed with the therapist who presented the case but one psychiatrist supported me in my view, Mr. E. S. was a paranoid schizophrenic. I suggested he be given nicotinic acid 3 gm. per day to lower his cholesterol (pointing out this would also remove his paranoid personality).

While in hospital he fell in love with an alcoholic patient who had been given treatment with LSD-25 as a psychedelic. She was then married to a psychopathic man from whom she had separated and intended to divorce. Mr. E. S.'s psychiatrist tried to break up the romance because he and other members of the staff concluded this romance could only be harmful to both. Mr. E. S. had also been separated from his wife because they were incompatible.

While in hospital Mr. E. S. reported that his daughter, of whom he was very fond, was normal but his son was a difficult and irresponsible alcoholic.

The discharge prognosis was pessimistic and the therapist reported to the referring physician that there would be no change in Mr. E. S.

The patient continued to take nicotinic acid (3 gm. per day) regularly, developed no more xanthomata and lowered his cholesterol blood levels to normal. He also remained free of spells and slowly found his personality began to change. He continued his romance; divorced his wife amicably, leaving her well provided for, and planned to marry again.

In March, 1960, he consulted me. Until then I had no personal contact with him and as far as I knew he had never been informed of any diagnosis. He knew that the nicotinic acid was recommended only to lower blood cholesterol which he knew it had done very effectively.

He asked me what was his diagnosis. I replied that in my opinion it was paranoid schizophrenia. He immediately relaxed, slapped his thigh and exclaimed, "I knew it!" He added that he had read as much material as he could get on psychiatry and had himself concluded he must have schizophrenia. He was not pleased with his tendency to view people with suspicion and wished to be rid of this symptom. The woman he intended to marry had described her psychedelic reaction and how it had been beneficial for her and he hoped I would let him have a similar experience.

Schizophrenia, uncontrolled, was one of my contraindications to giving anyone treatment with LSD-25, but, as he had been much improved for nearly two years and regularly took nicotinic acid in antihallucinatory doses, I concluded this could be done with safety in hospital. On March 22, 1960, he was given a psychedelic treatment with 300 μg of LSD-25.

The next day he was very enthusiastic about it, especially because he was able at last to describe the episodes from which he had suffered for four years. He said they were identical with some of the LSD-25 experiences. In other words, he had been experiencing minor and transient perceptual changes which were like the ones he had seen under LSD-25.

When free of his LSD-25 experience he completed two HOD tests (see Table I), one retrospective for his condition in 1958 and one for his present state (four weeks after LSD-25).

TABLE I

	Total score	Perceptual score	Paranoid score	Depression score
1958	51	18	4	15
1960	17	9	0	5

The patient has remained well and, as will be shown, was directly responsible for the successful treatment and recovery of his two children from his first wife and his daughter from his present wife. In addition, he has been providing help to a large number of other schizophrenics in his community.

In June, 1970, he was normal and I advised him to reduce his nicotinic acid to 3 gm. per day from 6 gm. to determine if this would maintain him. One month later he was moderately depressed and fatigued. His does was increased to 6 gm. per day which he will now take the rest of his life.

Mr. D. S.

Mr. D. S. (Mr. E. S.'s only son) began to develop many unreasonable fears at age 16. Shortly, he became an alcoholic. But he completed Grade 10 in school and worked with his father until he was 24. There was continual friction and difficulty between father and son. Mr. E. S., when he recovered, accepted responsibility for much of this. In 1959, Mr. D. S. began to drift from place to place and job to job—meanwhile continuing as an alcoholic.

Due to his father's persuasion he came for treatment of his alcoholism, expecting LSD-25. He was positive for malvaria, which is another contraindication for LSD-25 therapy. But because he had come a long way and had expected so much relief from it, he was treated on April 21, 1960, with 300 μg. Careful examination before this showed he was a paranoid schizophrenic with many visual and auditory hallucinations even when sober. During the LSD-25 session, he again suffered auditory hallucinations.

He was started on mega doses of nicotinic acid, 3 gm. per day, and discharged. He was somewhat better and remained abstinent for a few weeks but then reverted to his previous pattern. In my experience alcoholic schizophrenics are not helped by psychedelic therapy until their schizophrenia is controlled.

He returned for treatment of his schizophrenia in April, 1961, and was given six electroconvulsive treatments and his chemotherapy was adjusted. After discharge he continued to suffer many difficulties and consulted clinics and institutions in British Columbia. But since this discharge he continued to take nicotinic acid regularly and gradually continued to change his personality, repair his numerous marital difficulties and remained gainfully employed. In February, 1969, he became severely depressed and was given another series of ECT. Since then, according to his father, he was been well. His maintenance dose is between 15 and 20 gm. per day.

His HOD scores are shown in Table II.

TABLE II

	Total score	Perceptual score	Paranoid score	Depression score
April 1960*	42	6	6	16
April 1961†	92	19*	10	15
May 1961	67	9†	11	11
Feb. 1969	101	20	9	16

*Before ECT
†After ECT

Miss J. S.

Miss J.S. (born in 1927) was well until sometime in 1965, when she became depressed and fatigued. She was seen in the emergency rooms of the Department of Psychiatry by the psychiatrist who had treated her father. In his letter to her referring doctor he reported:

As you know very well, the whole S. family are pretty mixed up psychologically, although since Mr. E.S.' admission here in 1958 they have established a reasonably satisfactory modus vivendi. The compromise is based on each member carefully controlling feelings while recognizing the weak spots of other members. This need to bottle up her own feelings is inevitably taking some toll of Miss S. She is fearful of the impact of any argument on her father's health; she is fearful that they will die and leave her alone; she is fearful that they may have a serious psychiatric illness like schizophrenia and she herself may get it. She has very little in her own life which is truly her own and feels as a consequence greatly deprived. This was made much worse when he dog died some months ago and I suspect that this animal served a useful purpose in helping her to control her feelings.

I therefore advised her against the use of any medication directed toward the alleviation of psychiatric symptoms and suggested rather she get a new dog and begin to care for and worry about it rather than herself. I mentioned this to her father and I hope they will be returning home in order to get her a pup.

On returning home she filled the prescription by purchasing a dog, but there was no improvement. She was then given Trifluperazine 4 mg. per day by her family physician and recovered.

In the spring of 1966 her depression recurred and she was referred to me for examination, April 6, 1967. She complained of a persistent ringing in her ears; obsession with the future and what might happen to her family; difficulty concentrating and reading, and depression and anxiety. She was positive for malvaria. I diagnosed her schizophrenia and started her on nicotinamide–3 gms, ascorbic acid—3 gm. per day and Chlorpromazine—50 mg. per day. By May 4, 1967, she was nearly normal, and on July 28, 1967, was normal with only one fear—a fear her illness would recur.

She was seen again July 10, 1970, and was even better, stating she had missed no time off work, was sleeping normally, was not depressed and was free of all her former fears. In order to determine her optimum dose of nicotinic acid, it was reduced from 6 gm. to 3 gm. but after a few days her symptoms began to return and she immediately went up to 6 gm. She had not required any tranquilizers for three years. Her HOD scores are shown in Table III.

TABLE III

	Total score	Perceptual score	Paranoid score	Depression score
April 6, 1967	45	4	1	11
May 4, 1967	11	0	0	4
June 2, 1967	21	2	1	8
July 10, 1970	9	0	0	1
Normal Range	0-30	0-3	0-3	0-3

Miss S. S.

This girl was born in 1963 to Mr. E. S. and his second wife, both of whom had received pure LSD-25. She was physically and mentally normal. (In Saskatchewan there are no records of any congential abnormalities in children born to parents who had received LSD-25. From 1954 to 1970 more than 2000 subjects had received LSD-25.)

However, in October, 1968, this girl was referred to me because her parents were convinced she was developing schizophrenia.

She reported that every night she saw a large, white, tall ghost—as tall as her room. At first she had been very fearful of this but later she concluded that this was her mother walking through her room with a white sheet over her and there was no reason to be afraid. This ghost often spoke to her and told her she too would become a ghost. She also had visual hallucinations of many deer and foxes in her room. Her parents reported she slept poorly and was disturbed at night. During the day she played with several imaginary playmates whom she saw.

I diagnosed her schizophrenic and started her on nicotinamide 1 gm. each day and ascorbic acid 1 gm. each day. In a few months she recovered and has remained well.

Discussion

There is little doubt that the father and his three children are all vitamin B-3 dependent. One can rule out those vague factors such as faith, etc., which are so feared by psychiatrists and which comprise a new branch of psychiatry called placedology.

Mr. E. S. did not depend upon faith for he did not know me for two years, and did not know the nicotinic acid which he had taken for nearly two years might have an effect on his "spells." When he decreased his dose from 6 gm. to 3 gm. he had a good deal of confidence in me but still began to relapse.

Mr. D. S. had little faith in the medication but did take it regularly. As he began to improve his faith became correspondingly greater. Miss J. S. had little faith in the vitamins until she began to improve. After recovering, her faith was high. When the dose was reduced her illness began to recur. It is obvious that the placebo reaction is not dose-related. This dose response in Mr. E. S. and Miss J. S. is therefore very persuasive against faith as an important variable. Finally, Miss S. S. surely was too young to have any faith in any medication, nor did she believe she had been ill. This leaves the vitamin as the major variable.

There is no doubt this entire family once described as "psychologically mixed up" is now normal and none of the factors said to have caused Miss J. S.'s anxiety seem to be operative; Mr. E. S. is well and by no stretch of the imagination can be termed paranoid; Mr. D. S. is nearly well; Miss J. S. is normal and so is Miss S. S.

This family demonstrates the kind of family described by Heston. A superficial examination of mental state and an exaggerated interest in dynamics led to a diagnosis of obsessive compulsive state in a paranoid personality in Mr. E. S. and an anxiety neurosis in Miss J. S. Mr. D. S. could have been termed an alcoholic psychopath and Miss S. S. emotionally disturbed. But, if major perceptual disturbances (visual and auditory hallucinations) are basic in diagnosing schizophrenia as was described by Conolly and as many psychiatrists now believe, only Miss J. S. had none of these, yet all responded to megadoses of vitamin B-3. The speed of response was nicely related to chronicity. This is shown in Table IV

TABLE IV

RELATION OF RESPONSE TO CHRONICITY

	Age of onset	Chronicity	Rate of response
S.S.	5	Several months	One month
J.S.	38	2 years	Several months
E.S.	49	4 years	2 years
D.S.	16	14 years	5 to 10 years

Summary

A father and his three children are described. As they are all well while taking megadoses of nicotinic acid, they are diagnosed as a vitamin B-3 dependent family.

SCHIZOPHRENIA DURING ADOLESCENCE

Adolescent schizophrenia is often extremely difficult to diagnose. Adolescents are often labelled personality problems, adolescent turmoils, behavioral problems and so on. As the years pass it becomes clear that many of these children were, in fact, schizophrenic.

We think there are two main reasons for these failures to diagnose the disease early. Adolescence is a transition between childhood and adulthood. Most young people go through it without difficulty. But many psychiatrists have accepted the cultural myth that puberty and adolescence must be a turbulent period marked by many excesses of emotion and behavior. While adolescence may be a time of change and uncertainty, it is also a time of great hope and expectation when life is very well worth living. There is even some slight evidence that emotional upheaval is more frequent between the ages of twenty-one and forty-one.

The great majority of young people do not display unusual behavior during these years. There are fewer adolescents in psychiatric wards than one would expect from their numbers in the population. But if one were to judge from novels, plays, television and articles in national lay journals, it would appear to an interested visitor from Mars, who did not meet any of them, that nearly every young person is a juvenile delinquent or close to it.

But then, abnormal behavior is considered much more interesting than any other kind. It requires originality and even genius to write a play or novel about a normal child going through a quiet adolescence on his way to normal adulthood.

The unfortunate result is that, there is a tendency for psychiatrists to assume, when they see a disturbed child, that he is going through normal adolescence, but to a higher degree. The child's behavior and his relationship with his parents, brothers, sisters, teachers and so on are scrutinized most carefully, while the possibility that these may be disrupted by a devastating illness can, and very often is ignored.

The perceptions of young people are, in fact, less stable than those of adults. Boys and girls live in a very different world from that of their parents. When they are reading, lines move up and down and words may be blurry. This may have something to do with "reading problems" in primary schools. In adolescence, these may still be present, although the basic character of the young person is nearly formed.

We were only dimly aware of these striking differences between adolescent youths and adults until we began to use our HOD test. This test has been described in earlier chapters. It is simply a device which allows the subject to answer quickly a large number of questions about his relationship to the surrounding world. Many of the questions deal with the sensory apparatus. A scoring procedure was developed so that high numerical scores indicate the presence of much perceptual change. As we have said before, schizophrenics score much higher than normal people.

In order to understand the importance of high scores, we had to know what scores were common to normal people. We, therefore, tested as many normal people as possible. When we gave the test to adolescents between the ages of twelve and twenty-one, we were surprised to discover that a large number of them had scores which were in the schizophrenic range. Yet there was no doubt that they were not schizophrenic.

One of these was an intelligent young man of seventeen, with no psychiatric problems of any sort. He completed the test very carefully, and his perceptual score was high. He was questioned about each card and easily described the changes which he had indicated were present. We, therefore, tested a large number of normal young people in the city of Saskatoon, in Saskatchewan. Seven schools were sampled, using students aged twelve to nineteen. We found that the older the age group, the lower the HOD scores. In other words, the normal children aged thirteen had much higher scores than the normal adults, aged nineteen. If one drew a graph with age on the bottom base line, and scores on the vertical axis, it was nearly a straight line. The scores for each age are shown in the following table.

AGE	NUMBER OF STUDENTS	MEAN PERCEPTUAL SCORE
12	139	10
14	144	9
15	147	8
16	162	6
17	145	5.5
18	263	5
19	173	3
20 .	71	3
21-25	104	2
26 and over	99	1

But there are wide differences in the way adolescent students mature. Maturity consists in seeing the world in a stable way. We therefore define perceptual maturity as a lowering in the perceptual scores on the HOD test. But young people vary widely one from the other. Most adults, when well, are more stable, that is, they are more like each other than most healthy adolescents.

Not only is perceptual instability common in adolescence, but the ability to see and hear things in a stable way develops at different rates in different people. This explains why some adolescents have very low (adult) scores at the age of fourteen, whereas others have very high scores at the age of eighteen. We have also found that adolescents who mature more slowly than their mates are handicapped in modern schools.

When we examined all the fifteen-year-old students in one large sample, we found that those who were in grade eleven had much lower scores than those who were in grade nine. In the same way in the sixteen-year-old group those who were in grade twelve had much lower scores than those who were in grade nine. Intelligence alone was not the reason for the poor showing of the older students in the younger grades, since intelligence ratings are independent of age. Our perceptual scores decrease with age, but IQ does not.

We, therefore, suggest that perceptual instability in students is a handicap to fifteen-year-old grade grade grade grade school, excluding those who are ill. However, they will mature and there is no reason to suppose that they will then be worse off than others their age who go through school with better records. In fact, it is possible they will be more creative and productive, since some degree of perceptual instability seems to favor creativity.

Most adults forget the perceptual world of their youth. Indeed, what they accepted normally when they were young can be very disturbing in adulthood. If a fifteen-year-old normal boy hears his own thoughts (and many do) he will be little disturbed by hallucinatory thoughts coming from outside his head.

But at the age of twenty-five most people no longer hear their thoughts. Furthermore, they tend to forget that they ever had these experiences. If hearing of thoughts now occurs, it would be disturbing to the subject and he would make much of it for his psychiatrist. Unfortunately, most psychiatrists will not diagnose schizophrenia until they know visual or auditory hallucinations are present, and the schizophrenia of the fifteen-year-old has less chance of being detected than that of the twenty-five-year-old.

Whatever the reason, the fact is that too many adolescents are being treated for other illnesses when a careful perceptual history would have revealed they are suffering from schizophrenia.

If schizophrenia occurs during this period of life, the effect of the disease will therefore depend, among other things, upon the age and the degree of perceptual instability already present.

The first and most easily detectable change in adolescent schizophrenics will be in their performance at school. There will be an unaccountable downward drift of grades. A student who had A's in grades nine and ten may have B's in grade eleven, and C's and D's in grade twelve. The student himself may be perplexed and may work even harder, but he will find it very difficult to concentrate or read, and this will lead to a further decline in school performance. A large number of young schizophrenics from Saskatoon high schools have shown this downward trend in grades and have even failed. If the schizophrenic student is dull-normal in intelligence, there may be little change in school performance, simply because he is already getting moderate or poor grades, and the difference is not so noticeable.

Sometimes, but not always, the onset of schizophrenia is heralded by a marked betterment of school work. Students then become extraordinarily alert and creative, and do much better than ever before in school. But this is followed by the more usual downward progression. Whenever parents find their child showing such a change and can find no satisfactory reason for it, they should consult a psychiatrist who is not afraid to diagnose schizophrenia.

The second major early change is unaccountable fatigue. The students complain continually they are tired, will sleep much more than is normal, and will not awake refreshed from their sleep. This, combined with the inability to concentrate, adds to the difficulty of getting on in school.

These changes are followed by others, including perceptual, thought and mood changes, which are the same as in adult patients and have been discussed in previous chapters. But thought changes are more difficult to assess, for adolescents are usually more reticent about their inner world than adults. Since younger generations also tend to rebel against the ideas of their elders, the strange or bizarre ideas which may be the first signs of schizophrenia thought disorder are easily misinterpreted as signs of youthful rebellion.

A common mood change is depression, but occasionally the patient becomes overactive, together with an undue and tireless cheerfulness, punctuated by inexplicable outbursts of rage and sudden passionate weeping. This change is rare, but when it does occur it is a sign of schizophrenia.

The depression will be expressed in the usual way, with irritability or outbursts of anger. Several days of depression are often followed by several days free of it, only to be followed by depression again. Periods of deep depression often occur several times a day and are usually worse in the evening.

All these changes finally culminate in changes in behavior, and these can take any form. The variety of human reaction is enormous. The adolescent may become seclusive or act out his symptoms, or swing from one or the other. One of our young patients became sexually promiscuous and rebellious of parental authority, and remained so for several years. This was followed by the development of visual perceptual changes which forced her into seclusion. She was a very pretty girl, but now whenever she looked in the mirror she saw lines, wrinkles and bags under her eyes. Her face appeared so ugly she did not wish it to be seen by anyone.

She was diagnosed as an adolescent behavioral problem by a couple of psychoanalytically oriented psychiatrists who did not question her at all about her perceptual world. After nearly two years of psychotherapy she was ill enough to be transferred to one of us. Since then she has recovered with the aid of ECT (electric shock therapy) and nicotinic acid.

There may be increasing shyness, moodiness and an increasing reluctance to take part in normal social activities. Behavior becomes unpredictable. The sick child and the family are often only too ready to find some convenient reason for this altered outlook. At one time unrequited love was a favorite peg to hang it on, and Victorian novels abounded with heroines plunged into madness by heartless lovers.

One of our young patients was diagnosed by his psychiatrist as a malingerer because at school he gave completely bizarre answers to problems in arithmetic. It was assumed that he was trying to attract attention because his mother didn't understand him properly. He was given four years of individual psychotherapy by another psychiatrist and his mother was also seen many times. As a result, she became full of fear and guilt feelings, and he managed to limp along.

During the long years, more than a quarter of his whole life span, he remained moody, retiring, unpredictable, and troubled by recurrent periods of deep depression. He left home, entered the University of Saskatchewan, and a few months later developed a full-blown attack of schizophrenia with visual and auditory hallucinations. He had to be admitted to hospital for treatment, where he was given a short series of electroconvulsive therapy and nicotinic acid. He recovered, but he missed his year at university and has not gone back.

He remained well for several years while he continued to take nicotinic acid. But because he was so well, he stopped taking his medication and about six months later he relapsed. Again he was admitted to hospital where he once more recovered on similar treatments. He has been well for the past six years.

This case illustrates how schizophrenia, when improperly treated, prevents the unfortunate person from doing as well as his natural endowment would have allowed. Fortunately, this young man will do as well as his parents socially, and will not drift down the social scales as many other schizophrenics do. But it was possible to have diagnosed him correctly at the age of sixteen, since one of us at the diagnostic conference had then made the diagnosis of schizophrenia. Had the diagnosis been accepted, and had he been treated accordingly, he might have been spared two admissions to hospital, he would have completed his university education and his mother and family could have been spared needless guilt and anxiety.

Not every adolescent who suffers a personality change, fails in school and is troublesome, is schizophrenic. But so serious are the consequences of this illness, and so easily overlooked, that each case must be investigated for the disease so that early treatment can be begun. If it is present and properly treated, most young schizophrenics can be cured. If it is not present, other factors can then be examined and no harm will have been done.

Our malvaria studies showed that about one-third of the young patients under the age of twenty-one admitted to University Hospital were positive when examined for malvaria Of this group, those fortunate enough to have been given massive doses of nicotinic acid have responded well, whereas many of those who were treated in other ways have continued to suffer and to require prolonged treatment.

SCHIZOPHRENIA IN ADULT MALES

It is not possible to describe every form that schizophrenia can take, but by its very nature it is an extremely variable illness. We will, therefore, indicate some of the common consequences of schizophrenia in young men.

If it occurs before education and training are complete, it can interfere with, and prevent, the student from finishing his course. We, and many others have seen this in young schizophrenics, who eventually end up in occupations below their natural aptitudes.

One of our patients, now fifty-five years old, obtained his M.A. degree in history. Shortly after that he developed schizophrenia. Since then he has lived a solitary life on a Saskatchewan farm. He has been able to remain in the community because his family devotedly looks after him.

A very intelligent electronics technician had a brilliant future until he became schizophrenic in 1950. Since then he can only do simple farm labor, and only with careful direction.

With the knowledge we now have of schizophrenia, this waste of humanity is unnecessary. If properly treated, many of these young men will be able to continue their education and achieve what is possible for them. We have seen many young university students receive nicotinic acid treatment and continue and complete their education. We have today students and graduates in law, engineering, teaching, chemistry and medicine, who were once severely ill with schizophrenia.

The more usual case is that of a young man, married, father of several children, in a job or running a business or in one of the trades or professions. The illness may come on quickly and result in rapid effective treatment, or it may come on slowly. In the first instance, treatment is usually successful because the speed of onset focusses attention on the fact that something is gravely wrong with the sick person. There is no ambiguity or doubt in the minds of the family, friends and community, and the family are spared months and years of soul searching, trial and tribulation. It is, therefore, in cases of this sort much easier to receive the recovered person back into the family and community.

When the illness comes on slowly, the family must endure long periods of doubt, confusion and uncertainty. The ailing husband (his illness is yet unknown to the wife) becomes moody, irritable and fatigued, and now and then displays unusual ideas or behavior. This may shock or frighten the wife, but only briefly, for these are usually followed by periods of relative normality. But then the irrational moments become more frequent, more intense and last longer. The husband may become hostile and paranoid and direct this paranoia against the community. He is full of bitterness against his fellow workers, his employers and eventually against his friends. Finally he is irrational most of the time.

It can easily happen that the wife will accept his delusions as true and thus cease to be a bridge to reality, further hindering early effective treatment. For as long as she can maintain that his ideas are not true, so long will it be possible to maintain the patient in the community and delay coming to hospital.

Sometimes, however, a wife will mirror her husband's psychosis, and then we get a minor variant of a double psychosis. In one instance the suspicious and deluded husband believed the entire community was plotting against him. His wife was convinced this was true and the pair of them spent their days in a small apartment with the door barricaded against the world. Only his aged mother retained a link with reality and sought help. This wife was no help at all in getting her husband to treatment.

The suspicions may envelop the wife too and then her life becomes full of horror, for he suspects she is unfaithful, watches every move, searches for evidence to justify his delusions and indeed behaves very like Othello. If this goes on for a long time, the gulf between husband and wife may become so great that even his complete recovery will not help reunite them.

We have seen several cases where the psychiatrist treating the husband entered his delusional system and advised the husband to divorce his "unfaithful" wife, thus playing the part of Iago.

SCHIZOPHRENIA IN ADULT WOMEN

This is not much different from schizophrenia in men except that, since women have a different part to play in society, their illness has a different impact upon them. Because women are less often breadwinners, their illness may not drive them to seek help as quickly. For we tend to be much more tolerant of women who are poor and inefficient housewives than we are of men who are bad plumbers, doctors, electricians, and so on. The demands upon those women become less and less, their work is often done by husbands, mothers, sisters or even daughters, and so no one realizes how very ill they are.

Apart from this, schizophrenia in adult women is distinguished by two situations peculiar to women. The first of these is the period which follows having had a baby and the second is the period known as the menopause.

Women who are pregnant are not more predisposed to schizophrenia than other women. In fact, the opposite may be true. It is likely that pregnancy itself protects women against becoming schizophrenic. As we have shown earlier, the placenta manufactures ceruloplasmin, the protein which is successful in alleviating schizophrenia in many patients, especially if it occurs in women shortly after delivery.

The major increase in blood ceruloplasmin occurs in the last three months of pregnancy when the placenta is biggest. One might expect that some women might become better during pregnancy and in fact we have seen several women whose illness was much improved during the last three months of pregnancy. But it is not a panacea for schizophrenia for not every women is benefited and many who are, relapse after the baby is born.

Although childbirth and pregnancy are not especially danger-ous, nevertheless, there is a period for several weeks after childbirth when the danger seems greater. Women are not more likely to become schizophrenic during this period than women not pregnant, but most schizophrenic psychoses do come on within two weeks after birth. This should, therefore, be considered a critical time for women who have been sick with schizophrenia. It may well be that childbirth produces a false statistical increase in schizophrenia by decreasing the incidence for the last three months of pregnancy and by producing the especially vulnerable period for two weeks afterward. If one averaged the incidence over the whole year, however, one would find no increase in the schizophrenic incidence rate.

The content of the schizophrenia will of course be different, since schizophrenia in this puerperium period removes a mother from her family and creates many hardships for them. The results of treatment are every bit as good as for schizophrenia occurring at any other time.

The greatest danger here is that of incorrect diagnosis, for some psychiatrists, preoccupied with stress ideas and assuming the puerperium is very stressful, will only notice that the patient is low-spirited. Treatment for the disease must be started early and be carried on vigorously. We believe that nicotinic acid should be the main treatment supplemented with other treatments, and we have described this in Chapter V.

The question will arise whether the schizophrenia will come back with subsequent pregnancies. It may, but if patients are placed on nicotinic acid throughout the pregnancy, the danger will not be very great. Nicotinic acid is safe and has no injurious effects on the baby. Furthermore, the patient must be taught how to recognize her earliest symptoms and report them without delay so that help can be given. When this is done, the patient becomes far more confident and this in itself may prevent the possibility of a recurrence, or make it easier to bear by reducing panic and dismay. The patient should also be encouraged to keep in touch with her doctor day and night.

SCHIZOPHRENIA IN OLD AGE

The illness is no different at this time of life than it is during the middle years. The main danger is that schizophrenia will not be considered and that the changes will be labelled senile changes. There may be senile brain changes and the two conditions may be indistinguishable one from the other.

CHAPTER V

TREATMENT OF SCHIZOPHRENIA

PERHAPS you have been depressed for the past few months. For no good reason that you can think of you suddenly burst into tears, or you have moments of panic you can't explain. Your work no longer interests you. You are fatigued and miserable.

At the same time you may be having frightening experiences such as seeing flashing lights, noticing changes in people's faces, or feeling peculiar changes in your body. Something is happening to you and no one has been able or willing to tell you what it is.

Perhaps you are now taking tranquilizers and occupational therapy at a clinic? You are possibly making regular visits to your psychiatrist for deep therapy to "root out the source of your troubles buried in your psyche." Although you are willing to cooperate with your doctor to the best of your ability, you are frightened because you are not feeling any better, and you are convinced that you never will.

Or perhaps you have a close relative—a parent, or a child, or a sister or brother—who has, unaccountably, become very difficult to live with? Perhaps he has frequent outbursts of temper and moments of unreasonable suspiciousness? He sometimes says things which frighten you and does peculiar things which seem quite irrational to you. He may be receiving treatment for some vague "nervous" or "emotional disorder," but you have noticed little—if any—improvement.

What can you do now? Where can you go for help?

Millions of people all over the world are faced with the same dilemma you face today. There is nowhere they can go for information, and no one who can tell them why they feel the way they do, or what they can do about it. Mental health associations in England, Canada and the United States do not have any literature to which people like yourself can refer.

But for you, for your relative and those with similar problems, help is available. It is up to you to see that you get that help. We will describe here a treatment program for schizophrenia which we have developed and found effective in our own work, and which we think is the best available. We will furthermore examine what part other members of the treatment team—hospitals, nurses, family, community, and yourself—must play in this effort. For effective treatment of schizophrenia requires all the resources that can be made available to you.

Our views on treatment differ from those of many psychiatrists. Most of you, thanks to mass media, are already familiar with the ideas followed in modern psychiatric practices. But in the long run it is the public, you, the patient, and the relative of a patient who must decide whether a particular medical treatment is effective or not.

A serious mistake is to look upon schizophrenia as a "way of life" rather than as a disease. Medical men have a mandate to treat illness, but they do not have authority to tamper with a way of life. Those who do not think that schizophrenia is an illness cannot help the patient, and so should advise him to find someone who wants to treat him for his disease.

The next serious mistake commonly made is a failure to diagnose. Prompt and proper diagnosis is the first important step in the treatment of any disease. Without it, your doctor will not know what the trouble is, how to explain it to you and what to about it.

We hear a great deal these days about "treating the patient rather than his illness." This is nothing new. Many Indian tribes have long believed that confession of sins is necessary before the patient can get well. Witch doctorism, which specializes in driving out evil spirits, is related to this idea. Modern concepts of medical treatment, on the contrary, hold that we must treat the disease.

"Treating the patient" instead of the disease will often do more harm than good, for it frequently leads only to a failure to diagnose while the disease is allowed to run its course, crippling the patient and reducing his chances of getting well. Schizophrenia missed at the age of nineteen because of hasty or inept diagnosis, or because it was not believed important to diagnose, can lead to a lifetime of invalidism simply because the disease was not treated, and because the patient has not been taught the nature of his illness, or what precautions he can, and should take to assist in his recovery and prevent recurrence.

It is not unusual to see patients who are sinking into chronic schizophrenia while being zealously treated for a severe anxiety state. Instead of questioning the diagnosis, the usual explanation is that the therapist has in some way failed in his treatment or, more frequently, that the patient (or his family) is in some mysterious manner to blame.

But what has actually happened is that the doctor has not been able, or willing, to diagnose such a grave illness as schizophrenia. We cannot overemphasize, therefore, that when schizophrenia is present, it must be diagnosed for the very practical reason that we are advocating here: that if proper treatment is started early enough, the majority of the patients will be cured. Failure to diagnose schizophrenia correctly, in our opinion, is as serious, for example, as failure to diagnose cancer of the breast.

Research psychologists are developing other good objective tests of perception and thinking which may one day be very valuable. Projective tests, such as the Rorschach ink blot test, are of little value. Professor Hans Eysenck, of the Maudsley Hospital, Denmark Hill, London, has found them to be of no use and has presented a harsh scientific criticism of them. They have been repudiated by former presidents of the Canadian Psychological Association and the American Psychological Association, in the persons of Professor D. Bindra and Professor P. Meehl, respectively.

The HOD test is the only test that we know of which will not only help tell what your diagnosis is, but will let us know what is going on in your inner life in a direct and straightforward way. Even though we feel it can be much improved and amplified, we find it useful in uncovering changes in sight, hearing, taste and smell, and indicating what the patient feels about himself and others.

Without this simple yet essential information, we cannot begin to guess the kinds of troubles you will have, both at home and at work, because of your illness, and cannot help you understnad and live with it until you get well.

The test will furthermore tell when you are getting better and when you are getting worse. If we feel that you are best treated in hospital the HOD test is a valuable tool for measuring your progress while you are there, and will help us decide when you are ready for discharge, and show us during follow-up studies after discharge, if and when the disease is coming back.

In our preliminary examination we use the HOD test, in combination with the chemical test for one verifies the other, and the two together leave no doubt whether schizophrenia or malvaria is present.

The chemical test has the advantage of detecting the presence of either disease at a very early stage, and can lead to treatment at a time when the patient can still be cured. If you have the mauve factor in your urine, you have malvaria, no matter what other diagnosis you may have been given. Most schizophrenics have the mauve factor, but for reasons that we as yet do not understand, some patients who have the factor are not diagnosed as schizophrenic. While some may have been wrongly diagnosed, it seems likely that there are biochemical abnormalities other than this factor involved in the disease. The treatment, whether the patient has malvaria or schizophrenia, is, however, exactly the same.

Assuming then that you have found a doctor who has examined you for schizophrenia and has satisfied himself that you are suffering from this disease, what is the next step?

If you are sick, you must be told the nature of your illness and be given its name. You must be told, straightforwardly, "You have schizophrenia or malvaria", as the case may be. We find that the patient's response to the word "schizophrenia" will vary all the way from fear and denial, to marked relief. We have had a few who denied they were ill until they began to recover and realized they had been ill. It is, however, astonishing how many patients will take their medicine regularly even though they feel they are not ill. We have had several patients who diagnosed themselves correctly and merely came in to have this confirmed and to receive treatment. We have seen many who experienced a marked sense of relief when told what they were suffering from, for now they and their families had an explanation for their difficulties.

One of these was a very intelligent professional man who had been treated for homosexuality and alcoholism by psychoanalysis for two years. He was schizophrenic, and when told so, leaned back in his chair and exclaimed, "Thank God, now I know what is wrong with me." He was treated with nicotinic acid for several years, and during that time was seen a total of four times. After several months of treatment he married and is now a happy husband and father of a normal child. He is no longer an alcoholic and probably never had been an alcoholic in the real sense of the word.

This same sense of relief has been reported by many patients who have been diagnosed as having other very serious diseases, like tuberculosis, cancer or even leprosy. Almost anything is better than an unknown and unnamed ailment. Yet psychiatric patients are seldom told directly and simply that they are ill, that their illness has a name and that it can be simply and easily explained. Doctors usually evade answering such questions as, "What is wrong with me?" or "Do I have schizophrenia?"

One patient told us that his psychiatrist's refusal to answer his questions frightened him more than his symptoms. When he complained to another psychiatrist the latter said, "It's a good sign that you are angry with him," but did not explain why this was good. The patient later commented, "I was more afraid of what I didn't know than of my other fears."

Another schizophrenic patient, now fully recovered, reported he had several times asked his psychiatrist to tell him what was his disease. After one interview, he left saddled with an enormous load of guilt and frustration because no one would tell him whether he was sick or not. For how could he be sick if his doctor would not tell him the name of his disease?

Hallucinations are seldom attributed to the illness. Indeed, psychiatrists sometimes allow patients to believe that their hallucinations, illusions and other disturbances in perception are due to mystical forces, strange plots or the actions of the devil. To add to the confusion, some psychiatrists do not ask patients directly whether they are seeing or hearing unusual things, but make indirect remarks which are ambiguous and unclear. Meanwhile, the patient is not only hearing bizarre and often frightening experiences, but may be depressed, weepy and fatigued.

"I used to keep my white gloves clean all the time," one patient said. "I know they need to be washed now, but I just haven't the same interest, and no one understands. They seem to think I am lazy, or that I am pretending to be sick, or that it's all in my head."

A small matter? Not to the patient. Something is happening to her and she is not being told what it is. She wants to know what is wrong, but is allowed to go on living in fear and uncertainty. She has asked for help and is left to view the future with terror which the unknown inspires. She has no one she can look to for support, for she is quite uncertain whether even her own doctor knows what is wrong.

We have dealt with this in some detail because it is most important for the patient to know that he is ill, and to learn as much as he can about his illness. With the knowledge that he is sick comes a return of self-respect and a new status in the community, for it is perfectly acceptable to be ill. He can now accept himself as suffering from an illness, without harmful feelings of guilt and self-recrimination. He becomes subject to the old and complex rules which have been attached to illness for centuries. While others must show sympathy, understanding and tolerance, the patient himself is now obliged to cooperate in his recovery.

Many schizophrenic people are keen to do something about getting well. Harold is one of these. He will read anything he can find relating to his disease. He enquires about new treatments. He besieges social workers and others for any information they can give him. He talks about his illness freely. We consider that helping the patient learn about his disease, and teaching him to become aware of what he can expect because of it, is an important part of treatment. We tell our patients that schizophrenia is a disease in which biochemical abnormalities affect the working of the brain and produce changes in perception and other distressing symptoms. We discuss symptoms frankly. If, for example, you are frightened because objects appear to get larger as they get closer, a well-known but irritating symptom, or if you were to complain about extreme fatigue, we would then explain these as being well-known results of schizophrenia due to disturbances produced in the brain by the illness.

If you are suffering from delusions, we would tell you so and explain them as delusions. Some delusions are, in fact, reasonable but incorrect explanations for changes in perception, and they should be explained in this way. Many patients who fear that they are being poisoned develop this notion because foods taste bitter to them, and bitterness in our society is associated with poison. Few patients object to a frank discussion and many welcome a matter-of-fact explanation from a medical man who listens carefully to their complaints and is an expert on their disease.

No one must be blamed for your illness. It is common practice to blame relatives, husband or wife, or friends for the patient's condition. This is not wise and very rarely fair. There is little evidence to support the claim that schizophrenic patients become ill because their parents loved them too little or fussed over them too much. We do not believe that schizophrenia is caused by parental mistakes any more than diabetes is.

Psychotherapy of a deep and interpretive kind has not been shown to bring about any improvement in this illness, and many in fact consider that it disrupts the patient and may impede recovery. Blame can, and must, be attached directly to the disease where it belongs; it is enough for the patient to have to struggle with a grave disability without adding a further burden of guilt and hatred with dubious interpretations of an old-fashioned, psychoanalytic kind.

It is true that some close relatives of schizophrenics are themselves more or less ill. If this is so, then it will be necessary for the patient and the psychiatrist to decide whether it will be possible for him to live with them, then he will do well to part with them as amicably as possible. On the other hand, if he is going to live with them, out of necessity or for other reasons, it does not help to indicate to him, however lightly, that his parents may have deliberately driven him insane. Yet this has, in fact, been done due to an adherence to theoretical notions of a dubious sort. There are some gifted and brilliant psychotherapists who are extremely successful at making contact with very ill people by a variety of means. There are very few of these and most of those who treat schizophrenics are not in this choice category. It is wise to follow the old rule of doing the sick no harm.

Patients often make life difficult for themselves by alienating their family and friends with their peculiar or even repugnant ideas, and bizarre or unusual behavior. For this reason we would teach you not to act upon, or speak about, the peculiar things you may see, hear, feel or think. Some patients are surprised to learn that other people are frightened and repelled by their strange remarks and actions. It is not easy for them to understand that experiences which seem to be real to them are not shared by others, just as you may have trouble believing that a color-blind person does not see color the same way you do. Yet every day men survive by ignoring their senses. Disregarding one's senses is, we know, very difficult yet clearly possible. Pilots flying their modern aeroplanes are a common example of this skill. Our culture is one in which learning to disregard one's senses plays a large part in our well-being. Who would fly, drive a car, ride a bicycle if they took heed of what their senses tell them? Schizophrenics can also learn to disregard those sensations they know are misleading, confusing and wrong. But many patients have to be taught not to discuss their experiences with anyone except their doctor, their closest relatives or friends who have themselves had schizophrenia.

Even after their doctor tells them they are ill, some patients do not believe there is anything wrong with them. As far as you are concerned, it is not important as some doctors believe, whether you think you are, or are not, ill. Many psychiatrists consider that "insight" is necessary to get well, and that it is a good way to judge the results of treatment. Unfortunately, few of them agree on just what insight entails. Some psychiatrists consider that a sick person who blames his hallucinations upon a dominating mother is more likely to get well than one who doesn't. But there is no evidence for this. Insight can also mean having acquired the knowledge that one is ill.

We have studied the importance of insight, using this latter point of view, with a group of 270 patients. We have concluded that having insight has little to do with a favorable outcome. We found instead much evidence that those who did not believe they were ill were usually less sick than those who thought they were, and responded better to treatment. This is not difficult to understand. In less serious schizophrenic illnesses there are minor changes in perception, thinking and mood which are often harder to recognize than the more severe ones. Such changes may disrupt the patient in his home, work and social life, but will not be noticeable enough to warn him that he is ill.

In our view, then, it is much less important what you think about your illness than that (1) a proper diagnosis, using adequate tests, is made as soon as possible; (2) if such tests and full examination show that you have either schizophrenia or malvaria, you are treated properly for your disease; (3) you must act upon the advice of your family and your doctor even though your illness may make it difficult for you to do so.

It is not insight which is needed but faith in your doctor sufficient so you will cooperate in the treatment.

Finally, your doctor must know schizophrenia just as well as your internist must know stomach ulcers. He must discuss it with you in a manner that leaves no doubt about his knowledge and expertise, and explain to you exactly what treatment is involved, emphasizing that if you follow it faithfully your chances of recovery are very good.

Treatment Program

In the first edition of this book we referred to megavitamin therapy. But since our first book was written in 1966, there have been major advances in treatment. Much as cars made today are not the same as those made in 1930, so the present program is not the same as the one we recommended in 1966. For this reason we prefer to name our treatment orthomolecular therapy—a term coined by Dr. Linus Pauling in 1968. In an orthomolecular treatment program all the treatments in use today, i.e., tranquilizers, anti-depressants, ECT and other active chemicals are used but they are secondary or adjunctive to a proper consideration of nutrient therapy. This means that optimum diets are used combined with supplementation with vitamin B-3 (nicotinic acid and/or nicotinamide), with ascorbic acid, with thiamine, pyridoxine, and other vitamins which may be indicated. For each patient, once he is well, the non-nutrient chemicals (tranquilizers, etc.) are gradually withdrawn until the patient can remain well on nutrient and dieto-therapy alone.

We will not outline a complete prescription to be followed like a recipe since each patient requires individual attention. Professor Roger Williams has shown that individuals are biochemically unique. It follows that biochemical treatment must also be individualized. However, there will be sufficient information for physicians to become interested and for patients and their relatives to discuss it intelligently with their physicians. A physician's treatment manual is available from A. Hoffer, Saskatoon, Saskatchewan.

Our treatment program is divided into three phases, each phase depending on how long you have been sick, and how your schizophrenia responds to treatment. We will describe our rogram as if you, the reader, are a patient on the other side of our desk seeking help.

PHASE ONE TREATMENT

You have Phase One schizophrenia if you have been sick a short time and you are still able to cooperate with treatment in your own home. It may be that you are not sure you are ill or that you are unable to take your medicine regularly because you are forgetful. You can still be given Phase One treatment if you have someone in your family, or a friend who will remind you when you should take your medicine.

We suggest you take either nicotinic acid or nicotinamide* as your basic medicine, as both vitamins have the same effect on you. Both substances are B-3 vitamins; nicotinamide was once called vitamin B-3. Nicotinic acid (this is also called niacin) has an advantage which nicotinamide (also called niacinamide) does not have. It lowers the fatty substances, cholesterol and fatty acids, in the blood. These substances play a role in hardening of the arteries. Since hardening of the arteries (arteriosclerosis) can lead to high blood pressure and senile changes in the brain, it may be desirable to use nicotinic acid in cases where these additional changes are present.

We have to start with one. If we start with nicotinic acid you will be given a prescription for one month's supply at a dose level of three grams per day. They are available in one-half gram tablets. You will take two half-gram tablets after each meal. The first time you take them you will probably have a marked flush. About one-half to one hour after you take the tablets you will become aware of a tingling sensation in your forehead. Then your face will turn red and you will feel hot and flushed. The flush will spread down your body. Usually it will include your arms and chest, but very rarely will your whole body flush. There is no need to be alarmed. This is a normal reaction to this vitamin. There is no change in your blood pressure and you will not faint.

*In Canada and the U.S.A. 500 mg. (½ gram) tablets are available. These are preferable to 100 mgm. tablets since it is simpler to take 6 tablets each day and the larger tablets contain less inert bulky fillers. In Great Britain patients will have to make special arrangments with their chemists to obtain them in the ½-gram strength.

You will be uncomfortable the first time and you might be wise to take the first tablets in the evening while lying down in bed. Each time you take the pills the reaction becomes less strong and, within a few days to a few weeks, you will have become accustomed to them. Eventually as long as you take the medicine regularly, you will stop flushing altogether, or it will be so mild it will not trouble you. Some patients like to take the nicotinic acid right after meals.

Sometimes patients are bothered by the acidity of nicotinic acid. If this happens to you, you can take one-half teaspoon of bicarbonate of soda with the tablets. If, however, after you have taken nicotinic acid regularly as prescribed, and you are troubled by it, you may be advised to stop it and to take nicotinamide instead. Nicotinamide produces no flush at all, and for this reason it may be preferable for some patients. It does not lower cholesterol, but can cause some nausea.

The treatment you would be on would, in addition, depend on how old you are and what other physical complaints you may have.

For children, we prescribe 3 grams per day of either form of vitamin B-3. Children do not like the flush and it is difficult to persuade them to stay on nicotinic acid. They must stay on the vitamin until they are twenty-one years of age.

For patients aged fourteen to sixty-five, we prescribe either nicotinic acid or nicotinamide at the beginning. If either vitamin produces any unpleasant side effects, we prescribe the other. If you have a history of coronary disease, for example, or if there is a marked rise in blood cholesterol level, in your case we would prescribe nicotinic acid for it lowers cholesterol, reduces high blood pressure and slows up the process of hardening of the arteries. Or if you have a history of peptic ulcer we would prefer nicotinamide, but nicotinic acid can also be used for it can be obtained in a buffered form.

For all patients in this age group, we prescribe the vitamin for a year, and if the patient has a relapse, we prescribe it for another five years. We prefer nicotinic acid for everyone over age sixty-five because of its effect in lowering fat in blood.

You will continue on this treatment between one to three months. There is no point in taking smaller doses. If within this treatment period you show substantial improvement, then you will be advised to keep taking the medicine for five years when it can be stopped on a trial basis. If you remain well you will not need to start again unless the symptoms you had originally, begin to come back.

Patients who do not respond significantly are advised to increase the dose, which may go up in increments of 3 grams until a proper response is seen or until side effects are produced. The most common one is nausea occasionally followed by vomiting. This occurs at lower doses with nicotinamide. If nausea (or marked loss of appetite) does occur, the medication is stopped for one day. It is then restarted at a lower dose. In other words, it may be necessary to bump up the dose until nausea develops in order to find out the best maintenance dose. The dose will rarely be very high—up to 30 grams per day. When the patient has recovered, the dose is slowly reduced in order to find the best maintenance dose. It may be possible to reduce it to 3 grams per day or so. If symptoms recur, then the dose must be increased.

We also use ascorbic acid, beginning with 3 grams per day as a general supplement. Dr. I. Stone has shown that man cannot make any ascorbic acid and that if he could, his liver would produce about three grams per day when not stressed and a lot more when under stress. Dr. Linus Pauling summarized the evidence that these quantities of ascorbic acid decrease the frequency and disability from colds. Corroboration is coming in very quickly in spite of the general negative reaction of physicians and some nutritionists who have little experience with clinical nutrition. During a cold, larger quantities are used. Another indication is constipation. This in most cases yields to increasing doses. If the dose is too high, it will produce too loose a stool and the dose should then be reduced.

Another vitamin, pyridoxine or vitamin B-6, is being used more and more frequently, especially for children. There are a few children who do not respond well until vitamin B-6 is added to their program. Recently a hyperkinetic did not respond until B-6 was added to the nicotinamide, but by itself it was not therapeutic. Obviously, this patient was dependent upon both vitamins. The dose range varies between 250 to 1,000 milligrams per day, but one may go much higher, since it is also a water-soluble vitamin. On rare occasions B-6 increases irritability and restlessness, suggesting either that it is not required or that the patient is allergic to one of the ingredients of the tablet, which may or may not be pyridoxine. Other water-soluble vitamins which may be used are thiamine, or vitamin B-1, for depression in a dose range of 100 to 3,000 milligrams per day, usually under 1,000 milligrams, and vitamin B-12 combined with folic acid. The dose is determined by the response. Vitamin B-12 blood assays may be helpful in indicating when treatment is required and how much.

Other vitamins may be required. For example, Vitamin A for any surface lesions on the skin and mucosa (mouth, nose, etc.), Vitamin E (1 tocopherol) for aging patients or patients with vascular problems affecting any portion of the circulatory system, including the heart and the brain. The dose ranges from 400 to 2,000 I.U. or more per day. For patients who have had rheumatic fever it is wise to build up the dose slowly.

Calcium pantothenate or pantothenic acid are valuable especially for elderly people. This vitamin, discovered by Professor Roger Williams, increases longevity in animals, has anti-allergy properties and relaxes a few patients so they sleep better. The dose range is 250 to 1,000 milligrams per day or more. In some cases a multi-vitamin preparation containing most of these water-soluble vitamins is very helpful.

Just as it is important to give the most effective dose (optimum dose) for each vitamin, so is it important to give the optimum dose of non-nutrient chemo-therapy, e.g., tranquilizer or anti-depressant. Most psychiatrists are knowledgeable about these substances. The optimum dose must be that which controls or alleviates disturbing symptoms but which does not produce serious side effects, or immobilize the patient to the point where he cannot study, work or perform adequately in society. Sometimes performance may have to be sacrificed in order to produce relative comfort for the patient and effective control of symptoms. However, for every patient the final objective is a recovery sustained by nutrient therapy alone with the only occasional use of non-nutrient chemicals such as tranquilizers, anti-depressants, sleeping pills, anti-anxiety medication and so on.

We teach patients in this group, as all patients, to be alert for signs of recurring illness. We might tell you, for example, if you have dizzy spells, as you did before, or if you find yourself becoming depressed once again, or notice any of the changes of perception which you experienced during your illness, to resume taking the full dose of vitamin without delay. For the sooner treatment begins, the better chance you have of remaining well. If such a relapse occurs you should stay on the vitamin for at least another five years. We have found that very few patients get sick again if they take their medicine regularly.

Both nicotinic acid and nicotinamide are compatible with any other treatment you may need if you should develop any other sickness. For example, if you are pregnant you need not worry that the vitamins will harm your baby. Research with animals by our colleague, the late Professor R. Altschul, proved nicotinic acid did not injure rat infants. Recent work suggests that nicotinic acid given to pregnant women might have prevented their babies from being harmed by thalidomide.

But certain medicines are dangerous for schizophrenics and should not be taken. These are amphetamine, preludin and some anti-depressants. We have seen schizophrenia return because patients were given amphetamine to help them lose weight.

We encourage our patients to put on weight if possible, and do not allow reducing diets at this stage of treatment, because of the danger of relapse. One of our patients who began putting on weight as she recovered was placed on Dexedrine by her family doctor when she became twenty pounds overweight. The gain in weight was a good sign but her doctor did not know that, nor did he know the danger of reducing pills for schizophrenics. As a result, her illness came back.

Of course, as a patient on our treatment program, you will have had a complete physical examination. If your teeth are infected, you will have had something done about it. Any source of chronic infection should be removed or treated. If there are hormone deficiencies, this will have been corrected.

If you are following this treatment, and if your disease has been caught early, in all likelihood you will get well without having to enter Phase Two. If you have not made a sufficient recovery in Phase One treatment, if you have been sick for too long, or if your schizophrenia is so severe it would throw too heavy a burden on you and your family to treat you at home, you will be required to come into hospital for Phase Two treatment.

PHASE TWO TREATMENT

In hospital you will continue to take one of these vitamins as before but, addition, you will receive a short series of electro-convulsive therapy, ECT, for short.

ECT is popularly called shock treatment, but this is the wrong name for it. The patient does not have his sensibilities shocked, feels no pain, and suffers no loss of blood or decrease in blood pressure. In this treatment small quantities of electricity are passed across the temples. As soon as the current is started the patient falls into a deep sleep and then has a convulsive seizure, but he is no more aware of it than he would be if he were having his tonsils out. He becomes aware of his surroundings some minutes later, but it may take several hours before he is fully awake and alert. This treatment is safe, painless and one of the most useful treatments developed in psychiatry.

The word "shock," since it is misleading and frightening, is better not used because it makes patients and families unnecessarily afraid. Some have preferred to call it electrotherapy, or ET, and this seems correct, but ECT is more specific.

You will have anywhere from five to fifteen treatments, usually less than ten. The number given depends upon the response. It is given in the usual way with pretreatment with atropine to dry the mouth and cut down on excessive saliva and to ensure regular heart action. Just before the treatment a rapid-acting anesthetic is given intravenously, followed by a muscle relaxant. The treatment itself is painless and lasts a few seconds only. After that you will awaken slowly and will be somewhat drowsy until the effect of the anesthetic wears off. There are two kinds of treatment in use today: The first is unilateral, where the treatment is given to one side of the head only; on the same side as your dominant side. If you are right-handed, it will be the right side, if left-handed, on the left side. This treatment has many advantages over the standard or bilateral treatment. These are, (1) it produces less confusion and memory disturbance following the completion of the series; (2) therefore it can be used for outpatient treatment where admission to hospital is undesirable or impossible; (3) it can be given each weekday, thereby reducing the number of days required in hospital. With daily rates running close to $100.00 per day or more, this is an important consideration. This form of ECT seems particularly advantageous for depressions and for early schizophrenic patients.

The standard ECT is called bilateral. It is given three times per week unless there is a good reason for quickly producing confusion, when it may be given every weekday. It works best for chronic patients and should be used when unilateral ECT has failed to produce sufficient improvement. Both forms may be used; for example, bilateral on Monday, Wednesday and Friday, and unilateral on Tuesday and Thursday. Occasionally when a series of unilateral ECT has yielded no evidence of improvement after five to seven treatments, it may be desirable to complete the series with bilateral ECT.

Many patients are unnecessarily worried or fearful of ECT because they have seen it in movies or because they have read something evil about it; for example, that it is used for mind control and so on. There is no medical operation which is inherently pleasing to watch to the layman. If you watch someone having his tonsils removed you will not enjoy it, but this will not prevent you from having yours removed if they are diseased.

ECT should be given with the consent of the patient and it should be discussed in adequate detail to allay any fear. On very rare occasions it may have to be used without the patient's consent, and we have done so perhaps once every two to three years. In every case, the patient recovered, remained our patient, and was grateful that we had done so even against his psychotic will.

ECT does not damage the brain. The confusion and memory impairment go away eventually, although in some patients the memory of events occurring in the hospital never comes back or remains vague. This is unimportant as seldom does anything important happen here which needs to be remembered.

The megadoses of vitamins decrease the confusion and memory impairment and hasten the return of normal memory. In some cases we inject large quantities of these vitamins either before or after the anesthetic. This improves the quality of recovery.

We do not recommend ECT for schizophrenics unless the orthomolecular chemotherapy is also followed.

After the last ECT is given, you will be watched carefully for seven to ten days. If you have shown improvement, and if it continues after this period is past, we feel optimistic that it will go on for as long as you take the vitamin. Nicotinic acid or nicotinamide should then be continued for five years as in Phase One treatment.

In some cases, if we feel that ECT should not or cannot be given, we prescribe tranquilizers instead, but we use half the usual dose as the vitamin increases the sedative effect of the tranquilizers.

If you are cured with the combination of tranquilizers and vitamin, you will be discharged, and the tranquilizer dosage gradually reduced after several months. Our goal is to have you eventually get along on nutrient therapy alone. There are very few patients who cannot do so after such treatment. If the symptoms come back at any time during this period, we will increase the tranquilizer dosage, and try again later to reduce it until it is no longer required.

Most patients recover after Phase Two treatment, but some do not, and they then enter Phase Three when we add penicillamine, a breakdown product of penicillin, to the other treatment, together with a bit more ECT. In Phase Three about half the patients who failed Phase Two will recover.

PHASE THREE TREATMENT

This phase starts if you are not recovered, or not much improved, ten days after the last ECT has been given in Phase Two. We will then give you two grams of penicillamine a day for ten days, or until you develop a skin rash and a fever of 103°F. The fever may occur any time during the ten days and if it does, we will then stop the penicillamine. Usually the temperature will be normal next day.

If this allergic reaction does not occur, we will continue treatment for the full period of ten days. You would, meanwhile, be taking your full daily dose of nicotinic acid, and given three to five more ECT treatments. If you recover, you will continue on the vitamin as in Phase One and Phase Two.

If, after this treatment has been completed, you do not improve, it is because you have been sick so long that the disease has become chronic, and treatment will have to continue for a long period of time, either in hospital or at home. As a rule patients who have been sick for many years will not be helped with nicotinic acid alone. But if they can be improved in any way whatsoever, it is better to keep them on this treatment.

Finally, we will make every effort to get you well for no matter how sick you are, or how long you have been sick, you have a chance for recovering and we will not deprive you of this chance.

To do so you may expect many years of careful treatment. This calls for a lot of courage and patience on your part and from your family. Various aspects of the extensive orthomolecular program will be used, and you may require several brief stays in the hospital for addition series of ECT. Also you may receive large quantities of parenteral vitamins.

Chronic Schizophrenia

If the family can tolerate the patient's unusual behavior, and if they are able to live with him, treatment can be continued at home. It should never be given up too early. We have seen many very chronic patients recover after several years of such treatment. We have also seen many patients who were getting well suffer a relapse when doctors who were indifferent took them off their medicine or permitted them to stop taking it.

Mary Jones and Mrs. S. Brown (these are not their real names) are two of our many patients who are well today because we refused to give up hope. We have chosen these two cases to illustrate that every patient suffering from schizophrenia deserves a fair trial and treatment, that three to six grams of nicotinic acid or nicotinamide a day is effective treatment, and that a chemical treatment together with a carefully planned program for rehabilitation is useful in combatting the disease.

Both Mary and Mrs. Brown were given, by their own psychiatrists, little chance of recovering. Mary, in fact, was not only diagnosed schizophrenic, but retarded as well.

We did not believe that we could do much for Mary. We wanted to try to help her because we wanted to study schizophrenia at first hand and because her case was so severe it presented a challenge we could not ignore. And what better way to do this than to take her into our own home?

Mary came to the home of Dr. and Mrs. Hoffer after spending fourteen years in a grossly overcrowded, understaffed mental hospital. She was seventeen when first admitted, and had reached only grade four in special classes for defectives. Here she was one of over 1,600 patients. She slept in a large ward with 100 other women. She did not know what it was to have a place of her own to put a handkerchief, or keep a mirror. She had to stand in line to use one of the four bathrooms.

Little attempt was made at treatment. The hospital staff described her as impulsive, suspicious and quick-tempered. When she became violent and difficult to control, as she sometimes did, the staff had to restrain her or give her heavy sedation. She was often depressed and heard voices. While in hospital she required ECT and other treatment frequently, and after showing some improvement was allowed to do housework in the homes of staff members. She worked during the day in Dr. Osmond's home and eventually was discharged in the care of Dr. Hoffer.

There were three children in the Hoffer household. The home Mary came to was situated in a quiet, tree-lined residential street about two miles from the center of the city of Regina, and seventy-four miles from the hospital where Mary had been on unchanging routine for fourteen years. Mary had never been to Regina before. She had never seen a street-car or street-lights which turned now red, now green. She could not use a telephone dial and did not know how to take a message on the telephone. She did not know what to expect from the bustling household. She had much to learn.

When she came to the Hoffer household, a pale, dark-haired, dark-eyed and frightened girl, she was very quiet and did not talk. But she loved children and liked housework. She knew how to use a vacuum cleaner, dust, and wash and polish floors She was willing to work, was thorough and very efficient. Mrs. Rose Hoffer, with great patience, began teaching her the simple things she would need to know to get along in the city. How much fare she would need for the bus, how to count her change, how to get on a bus, how to use the telephone, how to buy a ticket for a film or do her own shopping. She progressed well for the first few weeks, and then became depressed and one day tried to kill herself.

One day Dr. Hoffer came home from the hospital early in the afternoon. Just as he entered his house he heard his son, age seven, shout downstairs, "Mummy, where is the electric light cord? Mary wants to kill herself." Bill was engrossed in a radio cowboy program when Mary asked him for the cord in order to kill herself and was too absorbed to realize the meaning of his message. Dr. Hoffer quickly ran upstairs and found she had the light cord wound twice around her neck and was beginning to tighten it. He immediately drove her to the hospital, angered and frustrated, having decided our experiment had failed. In hospital he gave her one emergency ECT because she was very disturbed. The next morning he told her she would be returned to the mental hospital. But she was somewhat better and wanted to try again. She was given one more ECT and that afternoon returned to his home. That day she started on nicotinic acid, three grams per day.

There were times when Mary went into fits of temper and brooding. The slightest thing at times unaccountably aroused her anger. Loud voices sometimes seemed to disturb and frighten her. Perhaps she misinterpreted a look or a word. But during the next two and a half years she improved to the extent that we considered her ready for discharge from this sheltered life into the community. Mary, we decided, had to be out on her own, working at a job and learning to be independent.

Dr. Hoffer found her a job as a cleaning girl at Regina General Hospital, and a light-housekeeping room close to the hospital. She would have to make her own breakfast, be at work at seven every morning, have lunch in the hospital cafeteria and make her own evening meal. There would be no one at her side to tell her what to do or how to do it. If she failed in her job, she would lose it. She was on her own for the first time in her life. Although Mary was frightened, she agreed to try.

When Dr. Hoffer moved to Saskatoon, Mary wanted to move too. They were now her family. Dr. Hoffer found her another job at a Saskatoon hospital. For the first few weeks she lived with a niece in Saskatoon before finding a room for herself. Finally, three years ago she found an apartment.

This story, we are pleased to say, has a happy ending. Any psychiatrist unaware of Mary's history would not call her schizophrenic or retarded today. In 1958 we began giving her nicotinamide when she complained of the nicotinic acid flush. At first whenever she stopped taking the vitamin her physical complaints and depression returned, but for the past two years she has remained well on no medication.

Mary is now one of the senior workers on the hospital cleaning staff and is efficient and reliable. Her income has risen steadily and she is completely independent. She owns her own furniture, including a TV set, manages her own money (a remarkable accomplishment when one remembers how incompetent she was with money on discharge from hospital), has money saved in the bank and has a reasonably active social life including boy friends. She is a girl of good moral character and has had no difficulty in her relationships with men. The efficient, self-possessed Mary we know today is a far cry from the frightened, uncommunicative girl who first arrived in Regina many years ago to try to live away from the hospital.

In 1991 Mary had retired. When she was last seen, in 1988, she was still mentally normal but was suffering from the earliest signs of congestive heart disease.

Mrs. Brown came to our psychiatric research service in 1958. By then she had been ill ten years, five of which she had spent in a mental hospital. For another four years she had required nursing care, with her husband and son looking after her. When we first saw Mrs. Brown, she was oblivious of the world around her. She seemed to be tuned in to a world all her own, with all contact with the normal world apparently broken. She heard voices speaking to her. Her thinking was completely disorganized. She spent most of the time alone, fiddling with her wardrobe, sleeping, or staring blankly into space. She passively did what she was told, and her speech was incoherent.

Mrs. Brown did not know where she was, and time, as we know it, meant nothing to her. She was locked in her own private world where she appeared to be living in a fantasy fairyland, saying that everything was very beautiful and wonderful.

We began treating Mrs. Brown with six grams of nicotinic acid, two grams of penicillamine and three grams of vitamin C a day, and ECT. After an allergic reaction to penicillamine, with fever and skin rash, she began to improve. When we finally discharged her, on three grams of nicotinic acid a day, she was much improved although she was not thinking normally. The family, however, was very pleased. For the first time in many years, Mrs. Brown, no longer a bed-ridden invalid, was cleaning, cooking and running the home well.

In 1960 she came back again, as sick as she had been before. We increased the nicotinic acid dosage to six grams a day and gave her another series of ECT. This time when we discharged her we arranged for her to come back to the hospital every two weeks for ECT, as an outpatient. Her husband gladly drove her the 350 miles for treatment. ECT stopped any further relapses and she has been making steady progress since 1961. Today she runs her household fairly well, knows who and where she is, is able to hold a normal conversation, and her husband considers it a pleasure to drive her into Saskatoon for follow-up ECT. She is taking nicotinic acid regularly.

Nicotinic Acid

It may seem odd to some people that a vitamin should be so effective against such a serious disease. The use of nicotinic acid is not an accidental discovery. Early in 1952 we began looking around for a treatment which would cure schizophrenia, assuming our theory was correct. An ideal treatment we decided, should be aimed at the biochemical process which was producing the schizophrenia but it should also be safe, easy to administer and cheap, so that patients could afford to take it for many months or years. Anything which would slow down the formation of adrenaline, we reasoned, might help. Nicotinic acid in the body can absorb methyl groups which are needed to convert noradrenaline into adrenaline. Large amounts of the vitamin would, therefore, prevent the formation of excessive amounts of adrenaline and this would slow down the production of the toxic adrenochrome and adrenolutin.

By the time we began considering nicotinic acid as a treatment for schizophrenia it had already an impressive history as a treatment for several delirious diseases. One of these is pellagra. Pellagra is a vitamin deficiency disease commonly found in countries where nutritional standards are low and people do not eat enough nicotinic acid. It was very common in some parts of southern United States before 1939. This disease was said to be characterized by the three D's: delirium, diarrhoea, and dermatitis. The delirium was very similar to schizophrenia. It has been estimated that up to ten per cent of the admissions to some southern mental hospitals were these pellagra psychotics. When nicotinic acid was added to American flour this psychosis was all but eliminated. This public health nutritional measure is the first major example of a preventive program in psychiatry.

Nicotinic acid had also been used for treating bromide-induced deliria, some depressions and some organic brain diseases in what was then considered to be large doses. We later learned to appreciate that these "large" doses were very small doses indeed, and decided to try it in more massive doses.

In February 1952, we treated our first case, a seventeen-year-old boy admitted to Saskatchewan Hospital in Weyburn with an acute schizophrenic illness which had started only a few days before admission. He was excited, overactive, silly and at times deluded. He responded only occasionally to ECT and was put on deep insulin, but this had to be stopped after less then ten days because he developed palsy in the right side of his face. During the next three weeks his condition deteriorated to the point where he required complete nursing care.

In May he was started on five grams of niacin and five grams of ascorbic acid divided into five daily doses. Within twenty-four hours he was better and ten days later he was described as almost normal. We stopped giving him vitamins a month later and observed him in hospital for three weeks before he was discharged to his home in July. A follow-up three years later showed that he was in good health, and had finished his final year of school. He has not been back in hospital since, and continues to remain well. He was interviewed as recently as June 1964.

Encouraged by the success of this case, we started our first clinical trial of massive doses of niacin and nicotinamide, using a placebo,* a sugar-coated pill, for comparison. We chose thirty patients from the psychiatric ward of a general hospital who were diagnosed schizophrenic by psychiatrists not associated with the research. We divided them into three groups at random, and started ten on placebo, the pill which would have no physical effect on them, ten on niacin and ten on nicotinamide. Neither patients nor the nursing staff knew which medicine the patients were taking; one half from each group also received ECT.

Of these, the placebo group did the worst. On the average, they were well only half the time for nearly two years after discharge. Patients who had niacin or the amide were followed up for just over two years, and they were well most of the time.

The success of treatment cannot be judged on length of stay in hospital since most hospitals today are making every effort to discharge patients into the community, cured or not. The criterion for effective treatment of schizophrenia is the same as the criterion for effective treatment of any disease: Does the patient get well?

The best way to determine the value of any treatment is to find out how well the patient does outside of hospital, and how soon and how often he needs to come back. This we did with a larger sample of patients. We found that schziophrenics treated in Saskatchewan without niacin or nicotinamide had a gloomy future; over half had to be readmitted to hospital at least once within five years of discharge. The niacin patients did better; only about a sixth needed more treatment in hospital during the same period.

One needs only to examine the figures of admissions to mental hospital, and compare them with the figures of first admissions, to realize that the treatments for mental illness generally in vogue today are not helping enough patients get well. In Canada,

---

*A placebo is a medicine which is supposed to be like the medicine being tested in every respect, but which is chemically not active.

United States and England, the number of re-admissions is almost equal to the number of first admissions.

Compared with these statistics, which one can find in any library and, bearing in mind that at present only half of the schizophrenics will recover whether they are receiving treatment or not, our own success with the vitamin as a treatment for schizophrenia was very encouraging.

In 1962 we followed up the first sixteen patients treated with the vitamin in 1952, and compared them with a group of twenty-seven schizophrenic patients who were receiving the treatments popularly in use at that time, psychotherapy, barbiturates, tranquilizers and ECT.

We found that the twenty-seven non-niacin patients did not fare very well. Seventeen of them, or almost sixty-three per cent, had to return to hospital for further treatment for a total of sixty-three times, and altogether the group spent thirty-four years in hospital over the ten-year period of this study.

By comparison, twelve of the sixteen vitamin-patients, or seventy-five per cent, did not have to return to hospital for further treatment, and are well today. The remaining four who did have to come back required a total of six readmissions for only brief periods, and the whole group between them spent only 1.4 years in admissions to hospital. None of this group are in hospital today.

To satisfy ourselves that our enthusiasm was not being conveyed to our patients and coloring the results, we followed up those treated with niacin by uninterested and even skeptical doctors while in hospital. Even these niacin patients did better. The results nearly five years later were similar to ours.

Other studies in our research program showed that the niacin group remained well longer than the non-niacin group. The results of one more study we did on schizophrenic patients treated at University Hospital in Saskatoon between 1955 and 1962 may illustrate the great saving made in human and financial resources when niacin was used.

Of the seventy-six schizophrenics given niacin during that period, twenty-one were readmitted for a total of forty-three times, spending 2,453 days in hospital. Four are now in hospital and none committed suicide. Of the group of 226 patients not receiving niacin, 122 were readmitted 275 times for a total of 25,341 days. Seventeen of these are now in hospital and four killed themselves.

Had the latter group been given the vitamin as part of treatment, assuming they were in no other way different from the niacin group, they would have needed only 8,520 days more in hospital, saving themselves a total of 16,821 days, and four more people might well be alive today. If we like to think of saving in financial as well as human terms, we can say that with niacin costing four dollars a pound, the outlay of two hundred and twenty-six dollars for niacin to get the patients well might have saved the Saskatchewan government $168,210 in costs of keeping them in hospital.

Included in these statistics are men and women who, except for their schizophrenia, had the capacity to work, were fathers, mothers, brothers and sisters who had something to contribute to society and who had the potential and the right to enjoy what society has to offer.

One of these was a young man whom we shall call Bill Young. Bill was admitted to a psychiatric ward in 1954 with repeated episodes of severe anxiety and depression. He was found to be normal in perception and thought, but very anxious and depressed. He was diagnosed anxiety hysteria and given intensive psychotherapy including interviews with amytal, the "truth" drug.

He was discharged improved, but anxiety and panic continued to plague him, and he was back a short time later with the same problems, except that he was, in addition, suspicious. In hospital, where he received psychotherapy, his condition became steadily worse. He lost weight rapidly. He began having hallucinations of sight and hearing, felt things about him were unreal and was obviously schizophrenic.

He was again discharged, but returned to hospital off and on until 1957 when he was diagnosed "character disorder and pathologic personality," a strange diagnosis in view of his symptoms. He was, nevertheless, started on nicotinic acid, which he continues taking to this day. He knows that if he stops taking the vitamin, his symptoms will return within a few days; his world will change, objects will seem smaller than they really are, and crowds of people will frighten him. Bill Young likes the life he has now. He is well adjusted in his job and is happily married and the father of two children. He has gained weight, looks and feels well, and is able to face every day with a good sense of humor and a feeling of well-being. He wisely refuses to go anywhere without his pills.

Without nicotinic acid and nicotinamide, Bill Young, Mary, and Mrs. Brown and many others like them would be in mental hospital today, swelling the ranks of the chronically ill in the overcrowded wards, hopelessly dependent on a society which is still looking for causes in the environment.

Both nicotinic acid and niacinamide are being used successfully today in Saskatchewan research in the treatment of schizophrenia. We have found that the treatment, which is safe and simple, can be combined with any other that the psychiatrist cares to use. If all medicines known were tested in order of toxicity, these would be found to be among the safest. There have been no cases of blood changes, allergies or other severe dangerous effects. There is only one case of jaundice reported in the literature out of many thousands of cases. We have seen none ourselves in over twelve years of treatment.

In view of the recent reports on tranquilizers, the remarkable safety and efficacy of our treatment program using nicotinic acid or nicotinamide becomes even more important. There is no longer any doubt that tranquilizers have improved the treatment of schizophrenia and that over the tested haul they are safe. A collaborative, nine-hospital study sponsored by the National Institute of Mental Health, Washington, D. C. examined several tranquilizers against placebo in a double blind study. Four hundred patients who were not chronic were tested. Among the group given tranquilizers three-quarters showed moderate to marked improvement. Of those given only placebo one-quarter were improved to the same degree. There were very few dangerous side effects. These patients were measured for improvement while still in hospital. It will require further follow-up studies to determine whether after several years the same results will be sustained.

Two Canadian investigators, M. M. Schnore and U. Kere, compared equivalent groups treated between January 1, 1948 and June 30, 1949 before tranquilizers were known, and between January 1, 1957 and March 31, 1958. In the second group nearly all the patients were given tranquilizers. Both groups were followed up four years. There was no difference in the number of admissions to hospital needed by both groups. The only difference was that patients were kept in hospital longer fifteen years ago. Thus it appears tranquilizers improve results in hospital but do not cut down the number of times patients have to come back for more treatment.

In 1957 it was not known that better results would be obtained if medication with tranquilizers was continued for a long time after patients were discharged.

But if this is to be done we run the risk of producing tissue damage in our patients. A. C. Greiner and K. Berry found twenty-one women who suffered peculiar purplish discoloration of their face, neck and hands. They had been given large quantities of chlorpromazine for three to five years. Of these twenty-one, twelve had severe opacities in the cornea and lens of the eye. Another forty-nine women had less marked skin changes. There is no doubt that many more changes will be found, for only now have these drugs been available enough years for these results to appear.

This, then, is our dilemma. Tranquilizers to be effective must be given many years but then the risk of permanent damage to skin, liver and other organs becomes substantial. We can get around this difficulty by substituting nicotinic acid for tranquilizers as soon as patients have made some recovery, for even after many years there have been no damaging changes due to it. If tranquilizers are needed, smaller quantities will be just as effective if the vitamin is also given. This reduces greatly the danger of dangerous side effects.

It may well be asked, if niacin is so good, why don't more people use it? First of all, few psychiatrists have heard of its use this way for the very good reason that it is a simple vitamin which is not advertised by any drug company; it doesn't belong to anyone in particular, i.e. it is not patented. No one is to blame for this, yet it has had a potent effect in reducing the information available about niacin. No one has had the financial incentive to draw doctors' attention to it or to have persuaded them to try it.

Secondly, as we have noted, it does not usually work quickly. It may take several weeks to several months to exert its full effect. In addition, these effects are seen to best advantage in studies lasting for several years. Very few studies of this kind are made in psychiatry because they are so expensive.

Thirdly, there is a bit of medical folklore that large doses of niacin are "dangerous." Accounts of just what the dangers are differs from source to source. None of these beliefs happens to be correct, for since our discovery with Professor Altschul that niacin lowers the level the cholesterol in the blood, thousands of people have been given these large doses for long periods.

Vitamin B-3 is indicated for a large number of other psychiatric and physical conditions. The following list will demonstrate to the reader the wide versatility of this powerful and safe vitamin.

(1) For depressions.
(2) For children with learning and behavioral disorders.
(3) For many cases of senility especially those caused by cerebrovascular problems. It is not effective against Alzheimers disease.
(4) It is an important component of the orthomolecular treatment of patients with behavioral problems.
(5) For arthritis.
(6) For hypercholesterolemia. Over the past five years it has become preeminent in this field following the final report of the Coronary Drug Study which showed that of all the compounds tested only niacin decreased mortality and increased longevity compared to placebo. It also elevates high density lipoprotein cholesterol, a property not shared with other compounds.
(7) Because niacin lowers histamine levels in the body it has useful anti-allergy properties. Guinea pigs pretreated with niacin did not die from anaphylactic shock according to Dr. E. Boyle. This was an experiment he conducted at the Miami Heart Institute when he was its director many years ago.
(8) It also has remarkable anti-stress properties.

Other Treatments

There are some treatments which may be useful some day, and some which are no longer in vogue.

Insulin coma was a very useful treatment at one time when no other was available. It is used very little today because it is more dangerous than tranquilizers and as a result has fallen into disfavor. We believe that many people, who otherwise might have become chronic schizophrenics, are leading full lives today because of insulin. Unfortunately, it was impossible to continue this treatment safely for months and years on end.

The relapse rate with insulin after three to five years is high and this leads some to claim that it was wholly ineffective. This was unfair, for one would not condemn penicillin because an attack of pneumonia developed months or years after the first one was cured. Similarly diabetics learn and expect to take insulin every day. Schizophrenia, which is a biochemical disease, does not resemble pneumonia and diabetes closely, but chemical treatment must be maintained for a long time, or until body chemicals are functioning normally.

In the past few years the importance of mineral metabolism has become very apparent, largely through the work of Dr. Carl Pfeiffer and his colleagues. As a result of these studies, Pfeiffer concluded that:

(1) Serum zinc levels of normal subjects decrease significantly in a six-hour period while copper and iron levels do not.

(2) Zinc, with or without pyridoxine, produces an EEG "anti-anxiety effect" in schizophrenics but not in normals.

(3) Urinary copper excretion in a six-hour daytime test period is consistently less for schizophrenics than for normals.

(4) Zinc increases urinary copper excretion as also does manganese, but zinc plus manganese in dietary doses is most effective in increasing copper elimination.

(5) D-penicillamine increases urinary excretion of zinc as well as that of copper. Therefore dietary supplement of zinc should be provided during D-penicillamine therapy.

(6) Approximately 11% of 240 schizophrenic outpatients had low serum zinc levels (less than 0.80 mcg/ml), 20% had elevated copper levels (greater than 1.20 mcg/ml), 8% had low iron (less than 0.60 mcg/ml), and 12% had high serum iron greater than 1.50 mcg/ml).

(7) The serum zinc or copper level may not reflect the tissue level since with Zn/Mn dietary supplements 50% of the patients had a rise in serum copper and iron over a period of 3 to 5 months.

(8) *Of the dietary supplements used in the schizophrenic outpatients, the best results were obtained with 3 to 6 drops of Zinc Sulfate 10% plus manganous chloride 0.5% taken morning and night.*

(9) The lowest serum copper level occurs one week after the menstrual period, while the highest level occurs the week before the period when women are most apt to be depressed. Estrogens raise copper levels and the schizophrenic appears to be more susceptible to this hypercupremia since serum copper levels of patients on the birth control pill may exceed those of the ninth

month of pregnancy. Hypercupremia can aggravate depression
and symptoms of disperception in the schizophrenic.

(10) Excess copper intake may result from drinking well water, use
of vitamin-mineral tablets, or the use of contraceptive pills.

(11) Other trace metals which have not been explored adequately
in the schizophrenias are manganese, chromium, molybdenum
and selenium.

(12) Because of zinc metal contamination (or addition in tablet-
ing) megavitamin therapy with niacin may in part be zinc dietary
supplementation.

(13) Those patients who have high serum copper levels, tremor of
the hands, ataxia and intermittent symptoms of schizophrenia
should be studied carefully as potential victims of mercury
poisoning.

(14) Analyses of hair shows male schizophrenics to be low in
manganese and high in copper. Females are high in copper.

A probable etiological factor in some of the schizophrenias is a
combined deficiency of zinc and manganese with a relative
increase in iron or copper or both.

Pyridoxine or vitamin B-6. Although our earlier research did
not include this vitamin it soon became clear in a few years that
for some patients it was as important if not more important than
vitamin B-3. Drs. Allan Cott and Glen Green found it extremely
useful for treating children with learning or behavioral disorders.
Dr. Bernard Rimland found it was the most effective nutrient for
patients having infantile autism. His findings were supported by
over a dozen double blind prospective studies. The dose range is
between 100 and 1000 mg per day with most patients requiring
between 250 and 500 mg. At these doses it has not caused any
toxic reactions. A few patients taking over 2000 mg per day did
develop reversible neurologic changes but the authors who
reported this finding did not describe what kind of diet they were
on or whether they were taking any other vitamins at the same
time. Orthomolecular physicians have not seen these reactions
perhaps because they seldom use single vitamins. Most often they
also use better diets and other B vitamins as well. Nevertheless
there is no need to go over 1000 mg per day.

Thiamin or Vitamin B-1. This water soluble vitamin has not
found any general use for the treatment of the schizophrenias.
However it must be used in treating the late stages of chronic
alcoholism especially Wernicke-Korzakov syndrome and it may

be helpful for some patients who have consumed excessive amounts of free sugars.

Ascorbic acid or vitamin C. We have used this vitamin from the onset but have not given it as much attention as we have to vitamin B-3. We were advised that it would be much more difficult to do carefully controlled double blind studies if we used too many treatment variables. We therefore decided to delegate vitamin C to a lesser role. However it has become more and more relevant as an anti-stress factor following the general principle that any disease is dealt with more effectively if that person is in a better state of health.

Our first patient to receive massive doses of vitamin C was a middle aged woman who had a mastectomy following which she became psychotic and admitted to the Munro Wing, Regina General Hospital, in 1952. After surgery she had developed a severe infection and her breast became ulcerated. The admitting psychiatrist diagnosed her schizophrenia and ordered electroconvulsive therapy to be started in three days. At that time I had decided to try ascorbic acid alone for a few patients just to determine what effect it might have. I approached the psychiatrist, told him of my interest and requested that he withhold the treatment long enough for me to try this out. I had planned on giving her 3 grams per day in three divided doses. He replied that he would delay it for another three days, and would start on Monday following the weekend. A.H. concluded that nothing could happen in three days with such doses and therefore ordered she be given 1 gram each hour, day and night. If she slept five hours the 5 grams would be given to her on awakening. By Monday, over the 48 hours, she had been given 45 grams. Her psychiatrist came in Monday morning preparing to give her ECT but when he examined her she was mentally normal and the treatment was cancelled and the ulcerated lesion had started to heal. She was discharged mentally well but died six months later from her cancer but she had remained mentally normal.

Another patient also responded to large doses of vitamin C. This middle aged woman suffered from severe depression because half her brain felt dead. She had never responded to any drugs or to vitamin B-3. The only treatment which gave her any relief was a series of ECT which would keep her well about 6 months. She would then return and beg for another series. About six years ago I advised her that I would give her 10 grams of vitamin C each day for a month and if that symptom was still present would then give her another series of ECT. At the end of the month she remained free of symptoms and told me she was going to look for work as a secretary. She has remained well.

It is now clear that we should have investigated the role of vitamin C much more seriously and carefully.

.

Diet and Other Factors

DIET

Schizophrenics tend to lose weight and to become thin and emaciated, especially during the severe phases of their illness. If identical twins are about to develop schizophrenia it will, as a rule, appear first in the thinner member of the pair.

If a patient is gaining weight, it is a good sign that he is getting better. When insulin coma was used more frequently than it is now, the patients who got well gained much more weight. For these reasons, a high-protein and high-calorie diet is needed. As long as a person is sick, he will waste tissues no matter what is done and there will be little weight gain until he begins to recover. Nevertheless, these diets should be continued, and after recovery an effort should be made to remain a little overweight if possible. A reducing diet is inadvisable, and reducing pills are highly dangerous for they may start the schizophrenic process again.

Dr. Allan Cott has introduced fasting therapy into North America after observing this treatment in Moscow several years ago. This is a hospital-based treatment, and requires special skill on the part of the therapist. After the fast is over, the patient follows a very special diet, low in animal protein. A few patients will undergo a repeat fast of one to three days at home every few months if they should notice a resurgence of symptoms.

Attention is also being given to special allergies. Some patients respond better to treatment on gluten-free diets or to diets free of milk, etc.

Finally, it is very important to remove as much junk as possible from the diet. We define junk as any food which is made from white flour or which contains added sucrose (white table sugar). The diet is high in protein (of animal or in some cases of vegetable origin) and very low in processed or refined carbohydrates. It is best for most people to start the day with a good breakfast and to have three meals per day with high protein snacks in between. These diets are described in several excellent popular books on clinical nutrition by Adelle Davis, Carlton Fredericks and others.

INFECTIONS

Any concurrent infections and other illnesses should be treated promptly and vigorously. Dosage of nicotinic acid or nicotinamide should be doubled until the physical illness is under control, for physical disease sometimes reactivates the schizophrenia.

SMOKING

Every time a person smokes, substantial quantities of adrenaline are released in the body and this is not good for schizophrenics. For this reason, schizophrenics should not smoke and should be discouraged from doing so. Smoking also depletes the body of ascorbic acid.

Brain Allergies

The megavitamin treatment has been evolving as more information has become available. This nutrient approach is more accurately described as orthomolecular therapy. So far we have described the way the vitamins are used, the importance of good nutrition and referred to minerals. There is a fourth component which has become increasingly important over the past year. Patients may be sick because their brain is reacting to a food to which they are allergic.

The schizophrenia we have described is a syndrome, i.e., it is a characteristic way the brain has of reacting to some disturbance in its operation. We believe that the majority of patients are examples of vitamin B-3 and vitamin B-6 dependency. The majority of schizophrenics are acute and subacute. They are the group who respond best to megavitamin therapy, groups one and two who require phase one and two treatment. A substantial portion of chronic patients (group three) respond very slowly or not at all. This has always puzzled us even though we were aware of the possibility they were schizophrenic for other reasons. Over the past year evidence has accumulated that a large proportion of these chronic patients are allergic to something in the environment, a food, or air-borne pollutant.

In 1962 Dr. T. Randolph reported at an International Congress of Psychiatry that he had treated 5,000 patients for allergy. Of this group 500 were mentally sick. When the substance to which they were allergic was removed they recovered. The introduction into North America of the fasting treatment by Dr. A. Cott awakened interest in the effects of food on mental illness. Several patients recovered by the fourth day of the fast. In the meantime Dr. E. Rees reported that many sick (hyperactive) children were responding to an allergy and became much better when they were placed on an allergy-free diet, and Dr. H. Newbold, Dr. W.H. Philpott and Dr. M. Mandell reported that a large proportion of chronic schizophrenics were allergic to many common foods, especially dairy products, wheat, corn and so on. They were able to cure by removing the food and reestablish the illness by giving it to the patient. This provided an explanation for the chronicity of the condition for the person is usually allergic to his favorite food and continues to expose himself to it every day or two and even more important explained why they did not respond as well to the megavitamin approach. Obviously one would not expect vitamins to overcome a brain dysfunction due to a brain allergy. One of us (A.H.) thus treated a series of megavitamin failures or partial responders with a four-day fast. This is a technique developed by Dr. Walter Alvarez, Dr. H. Rinkel and Dr. T. Randolph. The fast (and it may sometimes require more than four days) allows time to eliminate all the food from the intestines. The offending food is thus gone and the brain stops reacting and the patient will be normal or much better. If he is well this establishes that a food allergy was responsible. One determines what that food (or foods) is by adding one food per meal. When the offending foods are added the illness will reoccur (there will be a relapse) within one hour or so. This food is avoided thereafter. Over a four-month period 60 patients went through a fast, usually at home. They took no food, no medication, did not smoke but consumed 6-8 glasses of water per day. Forty were well at the end of the fast and have remained well since. They do not need any medication but must avoid the food to which they are allergic. The other twenty did not improve whatever.

The forty who recovered have remained well since. Thirty were allergic to dairy foods. Two were also allergic to beef. One was allergic to smoking, one to aspirin and the rest to sugar and other foods. Other orthomolecular physicians have found similar recoveries.

It is likely there are a number of reasons for the schizophrenic syndrome which may be classified in various ways. We suggest the following classifications: Schizophrenia is caused by:

A. Vitamin Dependencies
   1. Vitamin B-3
   2. Vitamin B-6
   3. Others
B. Mineral Disturbances
   1. Deficiencies, e.g., zinc, manganese, chromium
   2. Excesses, e.g., lead, copper
C. Cerebral Allergies
   1. Food
   2. Inhalant
   3. Food Additives

A rational treatment for schizophrenia is rapidly emerging and we look forward to a day when diagnosis will be quick and precise, treatment will be specific, controlled and effective, and when very few patients will fail to respond. The failures will be examples of cerebral disturbances of still unknown cause.

SLEEP AND EXHAUSTION

Lack of sleep itself will produce hallucinations and other symptoms commonly present in patients who have schizophrenia. Dr. Tyler in 1947, in one of the first experiments, kept normal subjects awake up to seventy-two hours. After thirty to sixty hours of being awake many schizophrenic symptoms appeared. They included increased irritability, lack of attention, loss of memory, illusions and hallucinations. Since then many other researchers have found the same thing.

If lack of sleep can cause normal people to suffer these changes, it is not surprising that lack of sleep, even though it is not as severe, can make mental patients worse. This is a common observation made by psychiatrists who work closely with their patients. In fact, patients are so sensitive to lack of sleep that many become worse from morning to evening. It is well known that physically ill people feel better in the morning after having slept. As the day progresses they become more and more fatigued until, in the evening, they may be very miserable. A substantial number of schizophrenic patients feel quite well in the morning but in the evening their symptoms can be most troublesome. About ten years ago we examined the nursing records of patients in the morning and in the evening. The nurses were not aware the study was being made. We were surprised how different the same patient appeared when the morning and evening periods were compared. In several cases a colleague examining patients in the morning could not believe they were schizophrenic. But a re-examination late in the afternoon dispelled his doubts.

Patients should be aware that lack of sleep can change them so markedly because this may have a profound influence on their reactions to their relatives and friends. Earlier in this book we showed how symptoms influence behavior. Lack of sleep or fatigue will increase these difficulties.

Schizophrenic patients often are not able to attend to the conversation of more than one other person. If they are engaged in conversation with two or more people, a powerful effort to listen and to understand, or comprehend what is going on is needed. This is easier for them in the morning. As a result they may drift away from groups late in the day when they will not do so in the morning. Recently we had a meeting with a recovered patient which required much discussion of important matters for several hours. After two hours it was obvious he was fatigued, much less talkative and had great difficulty following the conversation. This is not peculiar to schizophrenia. Other brain disorders produce similar changes.

Schizophrenics must ensure they get enough sleep. The ideal situation is one where they can sleep regular hours each night. Obviously there are times when it is not possible to do so. In this case it is a good idea to catch up on sleep whenever it is possible. The weekends are most useful for this. It is a good idea to sleep in late on either Saturday or Sunday. If the week has been especially fatiguing it may be desirable to spend a whole day in bed.

The bad effect of fatigue on group reaction can be reduced if patients are aware fatigue makes this more difficult. Patients should, whenever possible, make their major contacts with other people in the mornings and reserve their afternoons and evenings for private rest, quiet reflection or conversations with one person. If afternoon and evening group reaction cannot be avoided then patients should not hesitate to excuse themselves, leave the group and rest away from the group for a while.

Side Effects of Treatment

By side effects we mean unexpected effects of drugs or vitamins which are undesirable, often unpleasant, but which do not injure any organs of the body and do not lead either to death or permanent disability. Often the side effect is not caused by the active vitamin ingredient but by the other chemicals (like starch, etc.) which are also in the tablet in order to bind it into a useful tablet. Often the lactose or other sugars in the tablet are at fault. This is why tablets less than 500 milligrams in dose are undesirable.

The major side effects have already been mentioned. They are the flush, which is seldom a problem if the patient is forewarned, and the nausea. The flush can be moderated by using larger tablets after meals with a cold drink, or by pretreating the patient with an antihistamine. If the flush remains troublesome, it may be markedly reduced by crushing the tablets, allowing the crushed powder to stay in a few ounces of juice for ten minutes and then adding to it 1/2 teaspoon of inositol powder and allowing it to stand for another ten minutes. This also often removes the nausea.

Nausea can be dealt with by reducing the dose by 1 gram below the nausea-producing dose. If nausea remains a problem, it may be necessary to change to the other form of vitamin B-3. On occasion the dose of nicotinic acid just below the nausea-producing level is used in combination with the dose of nicotinamide which is below the nausea-producing level. This allows the total vitamin B-3 level to be twice the nauseant level of either one alone.

Nausea is apt to be worse during a virus infection. It may be necessary to stop the vitamin B-3 for a few days until the height of the viral attack has passed. If medication is not discontinued when the nausea is severe, it may lead to severe vomiting and dehydration. On a few occasions (out of 2,500 cases), this required intravenous fluids to control. In this instance a side effect could become a toxic reaction if not treated properly.

Contrary to the action of most drugs, vitamins have unexpected beneficial effects, or in other words positive side effects. Nicotinic acid lowers blood cholesterol levels and triglyceride levels which is generally very beneficial. It decreases the probability of coronary disease. Both forms of vitamin B-3 have anti-arthritic properties, something that many patients discover to their grateful surprise.

Other vitamins may have side effects as well, but fortunately they are usually minor and seldom are disturbing.

Tardive dyskinesia (t.d.) is a major toxic reaction to tranquilizers. For many years it has been considered irreversible by standard psychiatric treatment. Recent work suggests that it is not irreversible but when the drug is withdrawn it may after many years be cleared. The problem is that while it is going away the psychosis is returning once more, forcing the use of tranquilizers. It can come on within a few months of treatment and is more or less dose related. Patients develop uncontrollable muscular random movements which can affect any or all of the muscles. When the dose is reduced in order to decrease the severity of the reaction it may become worse. Mild or moderate symptoms will be tolerated fairly well but severe t.d. will incapacitate the patient. Several years ago A.H. saw a patient on parenteral tranquilizers whose whole body was affected. All his muscles quivered, twitched and jumped as if he were a bowl of jelly in a mild earthquake.

Tardive dyskinesia limits severely the use of adequate doses of drugs. It is also one important reason why patients refuse to remain on medication and have to be forced to take the drug by injection. Most relapses come when the medication is withdrawn by the patient or by the doctor. Drug companies are searching desperately for a newer drug which will not have this dreadful side effect. Clonazepine may be such a drug. It does not cause this side effect as frequently as do some of the other drugs but it does cause a different set of side effects and toxic reactions. One of the worst is a marked decrease in white cell count. Worldwide over 60 patients have died because of this. This is why in U.S.A. and in Canada the white blood count has to be monitored frequently. Sandoz was able to release it only after setting up conditions including weekly wbc counts. There have been no deaths reported in U.S.A. and in Canada. Its main indication has been patients who do not respond to very large doses of tranquilizers, i.e., without getting side effects. This is a rather heroic way of dealing with this problem while ignoring the fact that patients on orthomolecular treatment do not develop tardive dyskinesia. If orthomolecular treatment had become popular it is doubtful clonazepine would have come onto the market.

Dr. David Hawkins, one of the pioneers in orthomolecular psychiatry, reported that no cases of t.d. developed from an estimated 50,000 schizophrenic patients treated by orthomolecular methods. This confirms our experience on several thousands of patients. None of our patients developed this condition but we have seen many who were referred to us already having this disease.

The only effective treatments, apart from discontinuing the drugs, have been orthomolecular. Large doses of lecithin have been helpful in 40% of the cases. Had it been combined with vitamin C the results might have been even better as vitamin C helps regenerate vitamin E. Vitamin E, once a very unpopular vitamin in the medical profession, is now much more popular because it is an anti-oxidant and quenches free radicals; free radical theories are becoming very popular. The psychiatrists who have reported that vitamin E does help believe it does so by preventing the formation of free radical from the catecholamines, from adrenalin, or noradrenalin. However, they refused to name these oxidized derivatives as they are aminochromes. Adrenochrome is still a taboo word in psychiatry. These compounds or aminochromes are very reactive and can be very destructive in the body.

Neither lecithin nor vitamin E remove all the symptoms of t.d. This has been done by using a combination of manganese and vitamin B-3. This was reported by Dr. R. Kunin, an orthomolecular psychiatrist from San Francisco. But since manganese is not used routinely by orthomolecular psychiatrists, vitamin B-3 alone must have good protective properties. It may also function in this way because with the use of this vitamin much lower doses of tranquilizers are needed and may be reduced much more quickly. In 1952 we found and reported that niacin given by vein to epileptics whose electroencephalogram had been made worse by adrenochrome were made normal within a few

minutes of receiving the niacin. Niacin also protects patients with
Parkinsonism from the psychosis producing properties of l-dopa.

In our opinion the presence of t.d. in a patient is a measure of
the failure of psychiatry to use all modern information on
treatment and ought to be considered unethical. It contravenes
the use of informed consent. If patients were told they need not
get t.d. they would have a choice to use only drugs or to use
orthomolecular treatment. There is no doubt which choice they
would make.

The other main side effect or toxicity is little discussed in the
psychiatric literature. It is the tranquilizer psychosis (t.p.). This is
more serious for after it is well established it will be much more
difficult to repair, to undo the damage to the patient. Thirty-five
years ago Prof. Meyer-Gross in England described the action of
the newly developed tranquilizers as the conversion of one
psychosis into another. He meant that one set of symptoms which
characterized schizophrenia were replaced by another set which
he had not named. The basic disease process continued but was
much more subdued by the tranquilizer. This new iatrogenic
disease is the tranquilizer psychosis.

Readers of this book are by now familiar with the symptoms of
schizophrenia. To understand how these are changed into the
tranquilizer psychosis we will review the major symptoms and
how they change under the influence of the drugs. The symptoms and signs can be divided into "hot" and "cool" categories.
Hot symptoms focus attention on the patients and may force
them in to treatment in the community or into an institution.
These are the symptoms which cause major disturbances in social
relationships. The more severe they are the more intolerable will
be their behavior and the more quickly will they be forced into
treatment. If the behavior is primarily antisocial they will find
themselves enmeshed in legal sanctions. The most common of
these is committal to a psychiatric hospital. The other symptoms,
the cool symptoms, are just as disabling to the patients but do not
create as much social stress. A vivid example occurred many years
ago. A chronic schizophrenic patient was tolerated at home as he
sat quietly in his chair in the kitchen. However, a few days after
he began to hop up and down on his foot all day long he was
brought into hospital for treatment. His earlier psychotic behavior
resulted from his cool symptoms but his agitation and inappropriate behavior indicated they had become too hot to handle.

Hot symptoms are vivid disturbing hallucinations which generate inappropriate bizarre behavior. They are powerful delusions which also determine behavior. Fears and confusion are hot symptoms. Hypomania and manic behavior are hot as is agitated depression.

Most of the other symptoms described in this book are cool. In their presence patients and their families can carry on. They can be treated at home unless the symptoms become disabling and they can no longer be cared for. If they have no family, or support group, or shelter then cool symptoms can become incapacitating. The main advantage of cool symptoms, if they can be said to have any advantage, is that they can be treated at home, thus avoiding some of the dehumanizing effect of prolonged hospital treatment. The main advantage of hot symptoms is that they force the patient into treatment much sooner. With early treatment patients recover much more quickly on orthomolecular treatment.

Tranquilizers reduce or moderate hot symptoms but maintain or worsen cool symptoms. They create the new psychosis. This is not especially surprising since these drugs were originally selected because they were able to make animals catatonic. This is a peculiar type of muscular rigidity. The animals appear narcotized but are not unless a very large dose is used as is the case when it is necessary to immobilize large animals. Tranquilizers cause the following changes in symptoms

(a) In perception... hallucinations and illusions are dampened down but acuity of perception is decreased so that, for example, reading becomes much more difficult

(b) In thinking... this becomes more sluggish, there is more blocking, memory is impaired and concentration is decreased. Delusions may remain the same or weakened but the intensity of the reaction to them is moderated.

(c) In mood... this is flattened, less subject to mood swings and may lead to a general attitude of indifference. Joy and sorrow are not felt as keenly.

(d) In behavior... hyperactivity and agitation are decreased. Most patients become sluggish. It is more difficult to get up in the morning and they spend a greater proportion of the 24-hour day sleeping. They can be aroused from this sluggish state with some effort and can then function fairly well with simple tasks.

Because of their inactivity they expend fewer calories and may gain a good deal of weight which they blame on the tranquilizer. Sometimes tranquilizers cause a paradoxical state of intense agitation and hyperactivity.

This is the tranquilizer psychosis. Its main characteristics are hallucinations and delusions to which patients pay less attention, sluggish thought and difficulty with memory and with concentration, decreased activity, apathy, disinterest and indifference. This is why a person with t.p. can not function normally in our society. They can not practice medicine, fly planes, be plumbers, or secretaries, or farmers, or run homes, or do any job for which they could be paid. They can do some physical work under direct supervision but can not do jobs which require full possession of their faculties. In short they can not be employed and do not pay income tax. Tranquilizers convert hot symptoms into cool symptoms.

Tranquilizers allow the psychiatrist to move the patient between these two states. This is the nub of the tranquilizer dilemma for neither of these states is normal. With tranquilizers it is not possible to stabilize the patient at a normal level. Visualize two mountain ranges with a valley in between. One mountain range represents the original psychotic state and the other the tranquilizer psychosis. The valley in between represents normality. The problem is to move the patient from the schizophrenia mountain range down to the valley and to keep him there. But when only tranquilizers are used it is impossible to do so and they are taken back up to the other mountain range, the tranquilizer psychosis. In the valley of health attempts are made to keep them there by removing the drug, but then they in most cases are returned back to their original psychosis.

The only way today of keeping patients in the valley is to use orthomolecular therapy. Combining this with tranquilizers speeds up the journey to the valley. Once there the drugs are gradually withdrawn or reduced to such a low dose that there is no further difficulty keeping the patient there. The patient is at last offered a third choice, i.e., to get well. Orthomolecular therapy combines the best of both treatment regimens. Drugs accelerate recovery while nutrients maintain it. Drugs rapidly cool hot symptoms while nutrients remove all the symptoms, both hot and cold.

Toxicity

Toxic effects are those which threaten life or lead to permanent disability. It is not possible to consider toxicity without considering the toxic effect of withholding treatment. When a disease is very serious, as is schizophrenia, one is justified in using potentially dangerous treatment. When treatment is relatively safe, then it is in our opinion almost malpractice not to use it. The toxicity of drugs is described by referring to a therapeutic ratio. This is the ratio of the toxic dose, e.g., LD 50 (the dose which over a period of time will kill one-half of a group of test animals) and the therapeutic dose. If one unit is therapeutic but two units is dangerous, then the drug has a narrow therapeutic index. If the toxic dose is 100, the drug has a wide therapeutic index. The therapeutic index is very wide for vitamins. For vitamin B-3, the therapeutic dose for humans is 3 to 30 grams per day for nicotinic acid, and 3 to 6 grams per day for nicotinamide. There is no toxic dose for humans, since no human has died from an overdose or from using large doses. For dogs the LD 50 is about 5 grams per kilogram or about 300 grams per day for a 60-kilogram person. It is clear that the therapeutic index is satisfactorily high. For ascorbic acid it is even higher.

In sharp contrast, tranquilizers have a large number of toxic effects on every organ in the body. Schizophrenia is so serious a disease that this is tolerable, but it must be controlled by careful medical observation and control. Nicotinic acid, but not nicotinamide, has an undeserved and erroneous reputation for producing liver damage. This is not based upon any clinical data. This peculiar idea started with a study on animals over twenty years ago by biochemists who reported that it increased fat content of their livers. They did not examine the liver under the microscope. This study was repeated in exactly the same way by Professor R. Altschul several years ago. His studies showed (1) there was no increase in the fat level of the liver and (2) there was no pathological change in the liver when it was examined under the microscope. Psychiatrists are unaware of this work by Altschul.

In our own series of over 5000 cases, we have seen no cases with jaundice unless the patient was also on tranquilizers. These are well known to produce jaundice. A family physician in

Saskatoon who has treated hundreds of cases for over ten years has not yet seen a single case of jaundice in his series. If it does occur, it will hit fewer than one in 10,000 cases (tranquilizers do so in about three to six cases per thousand).

The acidity may be harmful for patients with peptic ulcer. They should buffer the nicotinic acid with baking soda and use the medication after meals only. The orthomolecular physician will be aware of the potential toxicities and will protect his patient against them.

Corroboration

Orthomolecular therapy is often said to be controversial. It is a very peculiar controversy, and non-scientific. Every physician who uses the treatment outlined in this book has been obtaining similar results. Orthomolecular physicians have little difficulty in giving their patients the individual attention which is called for. Because there are very few orthomolecular physicians, patients may have great difficulty locating one close enough to them. We are aware of a large number of patients all over North America who are being treated by non-medical professional people and even by recovered schizophrenics. They too seem to have little difficulty in following this program even though they are handicapped by not having access to prescription drugs, to psychiatric wards and to ECT. The orthomolecular camp includes a small number of world-famous scientists, a larger number of orthomolecular physicians and a very large number of patients in varying stages of recovery supported by their relatives and friends and by the schizophrenia associations.

On the other hand, the opponents of the orthomolecular approach include a few psychiatrists who have so far made no attempt to use even the most elementary approach, i.e., ECT plus megadoses of vitamin B-3, plus the majority of psychiatrists who have neither studied the program, nor attempted to use it properly, nor visited physicians who are using the treatment successfully. They have hardly any support from patients, presumably because their patients are not able to recover to the point where they could support any movement. We cannot imagine any tranquilized patients having enough useful energy to support any social movement.

Because of widespread publicity given to Dr. T. Ban's studies, we will refer to them briefly. Dr. Ban used only a combination of tranquilizers and nicotinic acid on a very small number of patients. In most cases they were chronic and institutionalized patients described in this book as phase two and three. They require long-term therapy with one or more series of ECT. This they were denied by the Montreal group. Dr. T. Ban is well aware of the fact that he has not done his studies properly and recently asked for our advice for a new series of studies that he plans to start. He now plans to treat Phase Three cases using Phase Two treatment. He still feels incapable of following our program. That is, he cannot start with a group of patients and follow our phase program as described here. There is an amazing reluctance to follow the proper orthomolecular approach. One of the reasons why psychiatrists are unwilling to repeat our studies is that they labor under the misconception that only double-blinded experiments are controlled experiments. Since we began the first double-blinded experiments in psychiatry in 1952, we have had over 20 years of experience with this technique, more than any other psychiatrist. We have concluded that this technique has very limited use, is very costly, very inefficient, and in our view is unethical, since it forces a physician to use drugs over which he has no control.

L-dopa, an excellent treatment for Parkinsonism, was shown to be inactive by double-blinded experiments.

However, agencies like the National Institute of Mental Health have forced researchers to use this dud technique by a too-rapid adoption of a method which has never been validated and which is based upon unsound mathematics, according to Sir Lancelot Hogben.

When establishment psychiatry shakes itself loose from its lethargy and uses the treatment as described, the controversy will soon be over. In the meantime, hundreds of thousands of patients are condemned to permanent disability by the unreasoning opposition of the professors of psychiatry who should be in the forefront in fighting schizophrenia.

Dr. T. Ban and Dr. H. Lehmann, his chief, never did complete their studies using what we then had called phase three treatment. But they did not rest there. Instead they spearheaded the American Psychiatric Association in its attack on orthomolecular psychiatry which culminated in the report issued by Dr. M.

Lipton. Dr. Lipton chaired a committee which was given the job of examining the claims made by orthomolecular psychiatrists and physicians. This they did by ignoring over half the reports issued by orthomolecular physicians, by ignoring all those doctors, and by highlighting a very few negative reports which made no attempt to repeat the original methods. The American Psychiatric Association Task Force Report On Megavitamin and Orthomolecular Therapy In Psychiatry, 1973, was criticized by Dr. Linus Pauling in his letter in the *Journal of the American Association of Psychiatry*, Vol. 131, pp. 1405 to 1406, 1974. He wrote, "I concluded that the general condemnation of the megavitamin and orthomolecular therapy by the APA Task Force is unjustified." Dr. Osmond and I replied to the APA in the brochure entitled "Megavitamin Therapy. In Reply To The American Psychiatric Association Task Force Report On Megavitamin And Orthomolecular Therapy in Psychiatry." This is available from the Canadian Schizophrenia Foundation, 7375 Kingsway, Burnaby, British Columbia, Canada, V3N 3B5. The APA has not bothered to reply, perhaps because they were certain their members would accept this report as the definitive conclusion and therefore they would no longer be under any pressure to read the literature for themselves. Unfortunately they were correct.

Problems in Giving Medication to Children

There are two main reasons why children have difficulty in accepting medication. Most often they do not know how to swallow capsules or tablets. Secondly, the tablets may taste bitter or sour. If the problem is one of taste, the medication can be made available in capsules. These have the advantage of being neutral in taste and they do not stick in the throat. Children generally prefer capsules to tablets.

If the child does not know how to swallow pills, then the medication will have to be given in a powdered form, which can be mixed with juice or (rarely) in the food. Nicotinic acid and other acid-tasting (sour) vitamins can be dissolved in liquid (not in milk), and if the acidity is a major problem it can be titrated with baking soda powder until the solution ceases effervescing.

This will remove the sour taste. Nicotinamide is very bitter and difficult to mask, but preparations are being developed which are overcoming this problem.

Children may be taught to swallow pills or capsules. One informant reported how she had trained her child. She crushed the tablets and placed the powder in the smallest available gelatin capsules. These are available in any drug store. The child had no problem. As soon as the small-size capsule was swallowed easily, she increased the size of the capsules until the child was able to swallow 1/2 gram capsules, which are available commercially.

With patience and perseverance on the part of the parent, any child can be persuaded and taught how to take the medication. Of course it is essential that the child be given an explanation which he can understand for taking the medication.

PSYCHOTHERAPY

You may wonder whether you will be given psychotherapy, since it has been so often repeated that it is the basic treatment in psychiatry. The best psychotherapy is given by a physician when he listens carefully to your complaints (symptoms), diagnoses promptly and accurately, advises you firmly of the diagnosis and then prescribes for you a treatment program which works. We will discuss with you whatever problems worry you, and we will advise you what is real and what is not real. When you are aware of changes happening to you we will expect you to bring them up for discussion. However, we will not give you psychotherapy which probes your past life, nor will you be advised to seek psycho-analysis, for these treatments have been proven to be futile for schizophrenia.

We will encourage you, as our patient, to study your place in your society. For schizophrenia produces difficulties for you and for people about you. Even if you are not fully aware of some perceptual changes we will explore them with you for they may profoundly alter your reactions to your family.

We have gone over the side effects and uses of nicotinic acid with you rather carefully. As a rule, patients who are so prepared, encouraged and given support will continue to take medicine until their doctor advises them they do not need it any more. They will not be worried by side effects.

We hope you will gradually learn to ignore perceptual oddities and to recognize them as transient recurrences due to fatigue when they do return. You should then increase the dose to six grams per day for a few days.

This then will be our form of psychotherapy. It will be rooted in the doctor-patient relationship in which you will feel free to discuss with us what troubles you, and you will have confidence in our advice about reality and how to overcome your perceptual difficulties and to reduce their injurious action on your relationships to your family and friends.

OCCUPATIONAL AND RECREATIONAL THERAPY

One day these forms of therapy will not be required, for every schizophrenic will be treated early and will recover. Unfortunately, too many patients have received treatment too late, or with too little skill. For them we require these additional aids.

EDUCATION

In most cases re-education is required. Chronic patients who have begun to recover may need re-training in simple matters which are most important. Patients may need instruction in up-to-date dress, how to apply make-up, cook, shop, use public transportation and other things he or she must know to get along and with which he may not be familiar.

The Treatment Team

THE HOSPITAL

It is quite possible that you will not have to go to hospital if our treatment program is started early. But if you do, what kind of hospital will you be in?

If you broke your leg, you would be going to a hospital you know something about. Perhaps you have visited friends there, or been in yourself once or twice for some physical ailment.

But as a schizophrenic you may not be so fortunate. Schizophrenics are often sent to hospitals many miles from home. You will be familiar with these as large remote brick buildings with many chimneys reaching up over the tree tops, far off the highway and outside city limits. The current trend is slowly swinging away from these large hospitals, and if it continues they will, some day, be replaced by smaller home-like hospitals in the patient's own community. A few such hospitals have already been built in Canada and the United States. In addition, more psychiatric wards are being built close to general hospitals.

Hospitals should be of the kind which will help and not hurt the patient. But few of them are. Within the past ten years studies have been made on the part that hospital design plays in patient recovery. It was found that there are two main ways of looking at a hospital. One way is to put more emphasis on economy, and we have large hospitals as a result.

These hospitals were built to hold up to several thousand patients at a time when the main objective of society was to get the mentally ill out of the way, and to save money at the same time. They were built to "store" patients in much the same way we store beer bottles. With this in mind we can understand why the wards were made very large, some of them holding up to one hundred patients, and why the corridors had to be very long. Since it was not known how to treat the mentally ill or what else to do with them, they were steadily stuffed into these institutions, many of which seemed about to burst at the seams.

It was also believed that the mentally ill lived in their "own fantasy dream world," where they were happy in their wild imaginings. A few patients, out of terror of shackles and other physical restraints, and unkind treatment, were violent and hard on the furniture. Why then bother giving them the ordinary comforts of life? Thus, in many large hospitals, one still finds a noticeable lack of attractive beds with spring mattresses and headboards, private rooms and private lockers.

The second approach is the ordinary ward commonly found attached to a general hospital. Psychiatric patients in these wards are separated from other patients by locked doors. These wards are generally attractive and comfortable. They have fewer patients per room and enough space per patient. They provide more of the necessities of life than the very large wards in large hospitals. Yet these too often manage to make a patient's life a little less than enviable.

Until a few years ago, these wards, like large mental hospitals, locked patients up "for their own protection and the protection of society." Any time a patient felt like leaving, he had to do so through an open window, although until recently there were bars across the windows also. Tranquilizers, plus more humane attitudes, made it possible to allow some patients greater freedom, and the "open door" policy was cautiously tried out in a few of the old-fashioned hospitals. When it was found to work out well, the idea spread to the smaller psychiatric wards.

The "open door" theoretically means there are no restrictions on patient movements. Many wards accepted the idea in principle, but retained the right to restrict patient movement whenever anyone on the staff felt like it. While doors were theoretically open, nevertheless the staff held a firm grip on the leash. When one ward in Saskatchewan was first opened ten years ago, for example, any psychiatrist who had a patient he thought might run away could say, "I want the doors locked today." So under the "open door" policy, the doors were locked ninety per cent of the time. Even today psychiatrists on some "open door" wards use excessive doses of tranquilizers to keep their patients so doped up they won't feel like running away.

Hospitals find a variety of ways of getting around the open door. We visited one large hospital which made no attempt at subtleties. One ward was open, but any patient who wanted to go out of that open door had to do so over the dead body of the guard hired to sit beside it.

Many hospitals on the other hand have no locked doors at all and these provide the most humane treatments. They have nothing to hide and are not ashamed to let the public in.

At Saskatchewan Hospital, Weyburn, one of the province's two large mental hospitals, staff members no longer dangle heavy key rings from their pockets since sixty per cent of the wards were opened in May 1963, by the superintendent, Dr. Fred Grunberg. The wards that are still kept locked include senile patients who may harm themselves by wandering away.

Patients on open wards in this hospital may come and go as they please, shopping or visiting downtown, as long as they remain within the hours set by ward staff. Those wishing to be out after hours may do so by special agreement. As a result there are fewer escapes now than there were when the wards were locked. In fact, in the early hours of one morning, an escapee was seen at a window begging to be allowed to come back.

This hospital is the kind a patient might not mind coming back to. In fact, sometimes when a patient gets a little out of hand, he is told he will be sent out of hospital if he doesn't behave. This threat usually works. Six years ago this was just another dismal institution for the patient who had the bad luck to develop mental illness instead of diabetes. As a result of extensive renovations undertaken a few years ago by the Saskatchewan government, it compares favorably, if not with the best hotels, at least with most modern hotels in any modern city.

The miraculous change came about partly because of public pressures, inspired by the Saskatchewan division of the Canadian Mental Health Association,* and partly because of enlightened superintendents and staff. It is an example of what people can do when they want to provide good hospitals for the mentally ill.

We do not imply that hospital design is the most important single factor. We believe that the standard of nursing and medical care is more important, and it is possible that patients may be treated better, with good nursing and medical care, in the worst possible wards than in luxurious rooms where untrained, incompetent and cold-hearted staff are in charge.

But we do believe that every facet of treatment must be maintained at the highest possible level. Unfortunately, hospital design has rarely been considered an important part of treatment for much of the last century. This is all the more surprising since the basic elements of design for housing schizophrenic patients humanely were clearly described about one century ago by Dr. Thomas Kirkbride, a famous American superintendent of mental hospitals. Mental hospitals have been designed as jails and as monuments. Governments who do happen to build a suitable hospital make use of it as election fodder over and over again before building another.

Patients who live in the hospitals are never asked what they find irritating about them, or what they like about their quarters. Nurses who work in mental hospitals are hardly ever consulted about the needs of their patients or asked how hospitals might be built to lighten the routine housekeeping load and so give them more time for nursing.

Psychiatrists are surprised if they are consulted. Even if they

---

*Unfortunately in the past seven years CMHA Canada has taken many aggressive moves against the orthomolecular approach by releasing partially false, and usually biased, information. They have deterred physicians from using the orthomolecular approach and have so condemned thousands of schizophrenic patients to permanent invalid status. The Canadian Schizophrenia Foundation was organized to do the job which CMHA failed to do and which was expected of them by the people of Canada.

are, there are hardly any architects who can talk intelligently with them—and *vica versa*—because their language and frame of reference are so different. Even when they do manage to achieve a useful interchange of ideas, it is the architect's ideas which usually find their way into the final design.

Fortunately, there are signs of change. One of our colleagues, K. Izumi, the Regina architect planner, has carried out extensive research into the design of the best kind of hospital for the mentally ill. It was not feasible for him to talk to patients, for those who live in hospital may be too sick to discuss function of hospitals, and usually if they leave the hospital they do not wish to have anything more to do with it. There was only one way he could find out what the patient's needs were, and that was to become one, temporarily, himself. By experiencing some of the patients' perceptual difficulties, he thought, he might have some inkling what problems the old hospitals imposed upon the seriously ill.

Mr. Izumi spent a great deal of time studying what mental illness was by discussing it with psychiatrists, and trying to understand the world in which patients live. Then he asked to be given LSD-25, so that he might see for himself what it was like to be mentally ill.

He took the drug several times and, while under its influence, went through hospital wards as he would if he were a patient. He noted the impact on himself of long corridors, of crowds of patients around him, and other features of large hospitals. At each step he discussed his impressions with one of us.

As a result of his studies as an architect and, briefly, as a patient, he concluded that patients would do better in small, home-like cottage-type hospitals, with only a few patients in each ward. He then designed new wards, in collaboration with Dr. Osmond, and these led to the construction of several new hospitals in the United States. Many of the Izumi findings are incorporated in a new mental hospital recently completed at Yorkton, Saskatchewan. The first reports from these hospitals have been favorable. They are considered by many to be the ideal hospital for the schizophrenic.

NURSING CARE

Nurses are important members of the treatment team. They need to understand what their patients feel, their pain, their altered perceptions and what effect these will have. Knowing what is happening to the patient makes it much easier for nurses to decide what to do.

If you were to suffer from delirium, for example, the ideal nurse would know it would be wrong to place you in a shifting environment, for this would only intensify your problems. She would understand your need for a single room with subdued lights, where noises are at a minimum and a quiet nurse is in attendance to provide support and help.

If you did not know where you were or what time it was, such a nurse would see the importance of making newspapers, calendars or a clock available to you. Visitors would further help keep you in touch with your environment.

If your time senses were distorted, she would see no point in saying to you, "Your doctor will see you soon." For to a patient with no sense of time passing, how long is soon? She would tell you, instead, "Your doctor will see you at three p.m.," or whatever the time may be. She would make a precise time statement and the doctor would have to make every effort to see you at that exact time.

If you are having trouble with your memory, she would expect to have to repeat statements for you over and over again. She would know she must act as another link between the reality of the average person and the unreality of the sick one, and not make vague statements.

If you have one or more delusions, she would in a matter-of-fact way make it clear this is an erroneous belief which you have only because you are ill, and where possible relate it to the peculiar perceptions which produce it. One patient was convinced that everyone with a name resembling Aly Khan's was after her. She used to get messages from the planets warning her about the deep plots being perpetrated against her. These delusions came from the distorted messages she was getting from her senses. An understanding nurse would know that humoring such a patient in her beliefs would only reinforce them and do her no good.

At the same time you have the right to expect nurses to treat you with the same respect as they would if you were well. This means that simple courtesies are followed. Mr. Doe should still be Mr. Doe and not become John as soon as he comes into hospital. We have observed that too often nursing staff look upon schizophrenic patients as childlike and, therefore, adopt childlike language and attitudes toward them.

Finally, nurses themselves can learn very quickly what your inner life is by taking one of the hallucinogenic drugs like LSD-25. They should, of course, do so under the care of a qualified doctor who is not an amateur with these drugs.

But they can learn as much, though more slowly, simply by being interested in these matters and reading appropriate books such as *Varieties of Psychopathological Experiences.**

YOUR ROLE AS A PATIENT

As a patient you have a grave responsibility to yourself and to your family to get well. You will have no problem if you are convinced that you are ill. But no matter what you think, you must do all you can to accept the statement of your doctor that you are ill, and of course you have a right to know the name of your illness.

You should be honest and frank with your doctor. Give him all the information you can about your illness and do not withhold any facts. But you are not obliged to tell anyone else about your hallucinations or delusions. As we have pointed out before, it is better to discuss some things only with those who you know will understand.

When a certain medicine is recommended, you must cooperate to the best of your ability by taking this medicine as prescribed for you. Some people are proud of "taking nothing stronger than aspirin." Some complain they are taking too many pills already. Either way, this is no excuse for refusing to take your medicine for you may be hurting only yourself. This attitude is no more sensible than refusing to take insulin when one has diabetes.

If the doctor finds it necessary to treat you in hospital, you must ascertain what your legal rights are before you go there. If you find these are infringed upon, you should spare no effort to have this situation corrected. Patients' rights are violated in peculiar ways and unless patients and their families do something about it they will continue to be deprived of their rights as citizens of their country.

*Varieties of Psychopathological Experiences, Fred A. Mettler, editor. Holt, Rinehart and Winston, Inc., 383 Madison Avenue, New York (1964).

Legislation about mental patients is apt to be peculiar and varies from state to state. In Quebec at one time, for example, in order to get into a mental hospital, one had to create a public nuisance on the streets, get arrested, be put in jail, and only then, if found bizarre, be allowed to go to hospital. In some parts of the United States, sanity hearings are required in court before one can get committed, and the presiding judge, himself a layman in these matters, makes the final decision, ignoring if he wishes the advice of a psychiatrist on whether or not a patient should be committed. Each state has its own laws on patient admission.

In Saskatchewan, as in the United Kingdom, the laws have been modernized to permit a patient to enter hospital voluntarily. One can also be committed here on complaint by a psychiatrist, a close relative or other responsible person before a magistrate.

A more understanding society is reducing the number of patients who have to be committed against their own will. Voluntary admissions are the best kind of admissions from the point of view of human dignity and the willingness of the patient to get treatment. The patient who admits himself voluntarily can discharge himself at any time.

All patients in Canada suffer a serious infringement on civil rights on entering hospital under the Federal Elections Act, which states that no patient has the right to vote while in hospital. Some professions approve, saying that patients must be protected from the "pressure" of having to make up their minds for whom to vote. This is nonsense. Patients in mental hospital should be allowed the same privileges of citizenship as anyone else, whether they wish to make use of them or not. If patients had the right to vote while in hospital, governments might be more careful how they treat them. Great Britain has solved this problem with the recent Mental Health Act.

But if you have a grievance you must be certain that it has a basis in fact, and is not a delusion resulting from your illness. To make sure that you have real cause for concern, you should discuss these matters with your doctor, who will be well informed on the laws and regulations.

Again we would like to remind you that you should insist upon receiving the best treatment possible. You should remember that your family is not to blame for your illness and should try to spare them as much trouble as possible. You should not blame yourself for being sick, but must accept responsibility for doing something about it. Your responsibility to get adequate treatment is greater than that of your relatives since it is you who are sick, and not they.

Your Family

The family plays an important role in the recovery of patients, for they have to bear the brunt of the problems presented by the sickness. The family's role will be discussed in three sections: before treatment is begun, during active treatment and after treatment has been completed.

BEFORE TREATMENT IS BEGUN

This stage is often the most difficult. The illness may come on in one of two ways, so swiftly that the change is obvious, or so gradually and insidiously that one is not aware of it until after it is well established.

If the change is swift it is merciful, for the patient himself either seeks or is easily persuaded to seek advice and treatment. If the illness causing the change is found to be schizophrenia, the patient and family are again fortunate, for then treatment can be instituted early, the disease has less chance of becoming firmly established, and assuming he gets proper treatment, the results of treatment are good.

Sometimes, however, the disease comes on so slowly that it is unrecognizable in the early stages. Only when looking back on it can most families realize how long it has been present. This sort of onset is most treacherous and holds many dangers for patient and family, which occur as follows:

Because it is not yet known the patient is ill, it is assumed he is bad-tempered, perverse, unreasonable, lazy and indifferent. Bewildered and upset by his strange behavior, parents persuade him to change his ways by berating him and showering him with rules of good conduct. Meanwhile, a disapproving community sometimes makes it plain that it not only agrees with the family that the patient is everything they say he is, but that it thinks the whole lot are at fault—the patient for being weak, and the parents for failing to give him the discipline and love he needed and still needs.

While the patient's illness progresses, the burden of guilt and anger in the family grows.

Everyone then applies sanctions or measures for suppressing bad behavior and encouraging good behavior. But the patient, the center of all this, is ill and cannot respond in a normal way. Punishment may be proof there is a plot against him and even kindness may seem to be a threatening blackmail. Because he is ill, he does not do as well at work or at school as others expect, or as he himself hopes to. Only when his behavior becomes bizarre, queer or irrational will the family realize the patient is ill.

One might logically expect that at this point the danger has been passed. It would appear that all that needs to be done now is get the patient to proper treatment, and all will be well. But it is not always as simple as that.

For now the family may be recruited as partners in the treatment, or they may be alienated, depending largely upon what the psychiatrist does and says.

The psychiatrist can help the family cooperate with him in a rational guilt-free way by telling them as accurately as possible what the problem is, and assuring them that they are in no way to blame. He can help them see the patients' behavior as being part of his illness and make it possible for them to withdraw the pressures they applied earlier.

Or he can endanger the patient and delay his recovery further by assuming the family to be responsible. This approach often precipitates another series of reactions which only add to the damage already done.

The first interview the family has, when a patient enters hospital, is usually held with a social worker. The questions the latter asks are designed to probe the patient's early life in detail. "What was he like as a child?" "Was he treated as well as the others?" "How did he do in school?" "How did he get along with his brothers and sisters?"

Rather than looking upon this as a joint discussion, parents might understandably interpret this interview as an accusation, and suspect they have somehow failed their child. This would be a natural reaction in view of the fact that parents are being held responsible for everything these days from bedwetting and thumb-sucking to car-stealing and schizophrenia. Seeds of self-doubt are being steadily and diligently planted in the minds of men and women who, sometimes through no fault of their own, become parents, and who, in most cases, are conscientiously doing the best they can in their difficult role.

Everyone, including chiefs of police ("parents are most often to blame for juvenile crime") to nursery school teachers ("we will teach you how to be better parents") have something to say about what parents must do to be good parents, and all have media through which to say it.

Since it is assumed in our society that parental neglect causes schizophrenia, therefore it is important for the psychiatrist to make it very clear early in his association with the parents, that they are in no way to blame. He must do this explicitly, and by implication. Relatives are often greatly relieved, surprised and grateful to find they are not to blame, and pleased and flattered to be invited to become part of an enterprise for helping the patient to get well.

If the seeds of self-doubt are allowed to grow, however, which they often are, they can turn into destructive shame, guilt and anxiety which may operate against the patient's well-being in one of two ways: the offended parents may turn away from the patient and his doctor, or they may take him out of hospital and away from active treatment.

We sometimes hear of parents who refuse professional help for their sick children, but we don't very often hear why. While the professionals have a soap box from which to expound their theories, the parents are seldom given an opportunity to tell their side of the story. And even if they were given the chance, who would give them a fair hearing? It is rather surprising that these parents, many of whom are intelligent men and women in other areas of life, have not yet formed an Association for the Protection of Maligned Parents. We recommend *And Always Tomorrow* by Sarah E. Lorenz (Hold, Rinehart and Winston). This book presents the parent's point of view well.

Very few doctors, psychologists and social workers seem to realize the shame, guilt and worry which build up in parents when told they are in some way to blame for the child's illness. The first thought may be to hide the patient and themselves from these accusations, and removal of the patient from hospital may be a natural reaction. This only adds to their unhappiness, however, for now their consciences bother them even more, making them less able than before to deal with the patient's disturbed behavior in the home.

Let us assume, however, that treatment is undertaken with the parent's blessings while the patient remains at home. What does the patient think about all this? He has been given a difficult time. His parents have been treating him as if he were bad, lecturing, punishing, cajoling for so long that deep wells of resentment have been building up inside. For a long time he has felt alone against the world. Suddenly he finds someone who is on his side, his psychiatrist. The psychiatrist listens sympathetically to his complaints and not only seems to encourage free expression of his anger, but may indeed demand violent verbal expressions of hate and distrust. The patient gladly gives him what he has asked for, but unfortunately, this unburdening does not lighten his heart. It only nurtures his hostility against his parents until it boils over into the home.

Instead of a patient being treated for a disease, now a home divided into two enemy camps—the parents, frightened and angry with the doctor, whom they no longer trust, perhaps even angry with the patient who has been causing them a great deal of trouble; the patient, resentful and angry, and not responding to treatment.

We have seen this happen over and over again.

Brenda Gallagher was seventeen years old when she first came to us as a patient. She had became a victim of an insidious form of schizophrenia beginning about four years before. During that time her behavior was such that her parents could only describe her as being immoral, difficult, unreasonable and many other things besides. It took them a few years to realize that she was not ill-behaved, but was ill. They then placed her under psychiatric care.

Her psychiatrist was well known to us as one dedicated to the idea that all schizophrenics are ill because their mothers or fathers had brought them up the wrong way, an idea still popular among some of our colleagues, even though the evidence for it is nonexistent.

She received psychotherapy, a "talking out" treatment, for many months, when she was encouraged to speak freely against her parents, and to talk about any problems she could bring to mind. For six months more, in hospital, she was treated with permissive psychotherapy. Instead of getting better, she got worse. Her behavior, which before was merely bad, was now intolerable. She was then transferred to our care as a last resort before committing her.*

In our first interview, we informed her for the first time that she was ill, that she had schizophrenia and that she would be treated with nicotinic acid plus ECT. She spoke very angrily about her parents whom she blamed for her difficulties. We told her that they were in no way responsible for her illness.

She was treated for some months in this way, and began making great improvement. When she was discharged, her relations with her parents were good and she no longer voiced her delusional hostility against them. She has remained well for nearly six years without requiring further treatment. And she gets along well with her parents.

AFTER TREATMENT HAS STARTED

Once treatment has started, it is the job of all relatives to see that everything is being done to help the patient get well.

If the patient receives treatment at home, all his family must accept the fact that he is ill and be as considerate and cooperative as possible. They must help him decide what is real and what is not real. They must make it clear to the patient that they love and trust him, no matter what he might think at times, that they are trying to help him in every way possible and that they are making an effort to understand how he feels. They must act as a link between him and the community, at the same time making it clear to the community that he is ill and not the perverse person he is considered to be.

If treatment is given in hospital, relatives should visit frequently, bringing him news from home, school or friends. If visiting is impossible they should write, telephone or in other ways show their affection and concern. They should not make promises to visit which they cannot keep. When they see the patient they should be interested in what he has to say and remain calm and reassuring. If the patient is confused because of ECT or drug treatment, they should reassure him that this is part of getting well.

Maintaining this attention will be most difficult when patients must be treated in hospital from several months to several years. But relatives must not lose interest or drift away.

Patients are very often too sick to speak for themselves. If hospitals are overcrowded, show lack of concern in any way, and treat patients as though they are somewhat less than human, they should not be put off merely by statements that schizophrenia is this or that which prevents better care.

Some doctors and nurses once had, and still have, fantastic notions about schizophrenia. They may believe, for instance, as many once did, that if schizophrenics refuse to wear clothes it is because it is in the nature of some schizophrenics not to wear clothes. This is nonsense. It is in the nature of schizophrenics to be ill. If they will not wear clothes it is because there has been a complete misunderstanding among hospital staff how to treat them.

In badly run hospitals, patients look shabby, dilapidated and even ragged. In well-run hospitals they may look ill and unhappy, as they often are, but they are dressed like everyone else, so that they need not feel ashamed or degraded when they begin getting better. In the Weyburn Hospital it is often difficult to tell patients from visitors. Most women patients wear make-up and their hair is neatly kept. All patients are allowed to wear the clothes they bring with them.

It may be that in some hospitals the clothing is of such quality and style that even a normal person might prefer to be nude rather than wear it. It could even be that clothes are not provided often enough. Properly run hospitals have no patients who refuse to wear clothes.

It is a relative's duty and right to insist that the hospital the patient is in now is as good as the hospital he was in when he had his appendix out. They must demand that it is the kind of hospital that will help and not hurt him, and that it will not add to the feeling of disgrace presently attached to the disease called schizophrenia.

If the hospital is not doing its job—and its job is to give the patient the best possible care in pleasant, attractive surround-ings—the relatives should make this emphatically known to their doctor, to the hospital superintendent, to their senators, congress-men, members of parliament, civic officials and anyone else in a position to do something about it.

Relatives must not accept the often spurious claim that the government is giving the patient better care than he would be getting somewhere else. Governments like to deal with statistics which show that their mental health program is better than the mental health program of any other government. This is not good enough. Relatives should demand that the care is as good as the care given to a neighbor who is in hospital with a duodenal ulcer.

A patient's relatives should, furthermore, be skeptical of the claim that governments are looking after all the needs of the mentally ill. If they were, there would be no need for mental health associations. Many of these are filling the gap in mental health services by providing rehabilitation services not given by governments, such as White Cross centers being operated by the Canadian Mental Health Association. A relative can make his wishes known by supporting such an organization and seeing to it that it exerts pressure on reluctant governments on behalf of the mentally ill. Only when legislators realize that for each patient in hospital there are two or more ex-patients outside who vote, and numerous concerned relatives who support them, will there be a great change in mental hospitals.

AFTER DISCHARGE

Well, now the patient is home from hospital. Relatives should continue to cooperate with the treatment, seeing to it that the discharged patient takes his medicine regularly, gets enough sleep and so on. They might have to bear with him for a while, for his behavior might still demand patience. However, as he recovers, more can be expected of him and he can gradually be treated as any normal individual. It must now be accepted that his illness has been in the past, and his behavior must be forgotten. He must be accepted as he is now and not as he was before.

His past illness must never be used as a weapon against him, or to make him feel inferior. For a relative must remember that his own genes are the same as the patient's, but that the latter was ill because he happened to get a larger number of certain genes or inherited factors. This does not make him inferior any more than it makes a sane relative superior.

The Community

The community has responsibilities no less important than the patients' and their families'. Unfortunately, it does not often realize it. It is said that no community is stronger than its weakest link. The effects of illness in one individual involve other members in ever-widening circles until everyone is directly or indirectly enmeshed.

Whole systems have been devised to pick up the pieces after sick members in our communities—jails, police courts, police; welfare agencies including social aid; heavily staffed civil servant organizations; private organizations, some of which are effective in planning their programs to encourage cure and rehabilitation, and some of which are ineffective, ignoring causes and treatment.

The trend seems to be to shift treatment responsibility to the community because psychiatrists do not know how to cure the mentally ill. More home care is needed because more patients are being discharged, yet they are not being cured. Better treatment would result in less time spent in hospital and less suffering and shame. It would make rehabilitation less essential and reduce the demands on the community.

The responsibility of the community is to:

1. Provide adequate hospitals.

2. Staff them with competent psychiatrists and adequate professional staff.

3. Encourage and demand effective treatment of the sick.

4. Accept them back as soon as they are ready without attaching any stigma to them, and help to rehabilitate them by providing jobs and homes.

5. Above all, support research which will give us answers to puzzling questions. When this is done, there will be a noticeable reduction in the efforts we must now make and the money we must now spend to endure sick people who have not been helped.

On the basis of clinical experience by A.H. accumulated since 1955 the following treatment results will be obtained by any physician following the program outline in this volume and also in *Orthomolecular Medicine for Physicians*, by A. Hoffer, Keats Publishing, Inc. New Canaan, Conn, U.S.A. 1989.

TABLE SHOWING THE RESULTS OF TREATMENT
USING ORTHOMOLECULAR METHODS

Group	Duration of treatment	Well and Much Improved
Sick one year or in second or third relapse	Up to one year	90%

Sick two to five years	Up to five years	75%
Sick over five years, out of hospital	Five or more years	50%
Sick over five years, in hospital	Five or more years	25%

These results are better than those obtained by using tranquilizers alone. In fact, it is not possible to recover and to stay well on tranquilizers alone. This has been examined in some detail in the section on side effects.

CHAPTER VI

PREVENTING SCHIZOPHRENIA

THIS will be a very short chapter for at present we do not know how to prevent schizophrenia. One cannot prevent until one is able to predict.

We can predict, for example that chlorinating drinking water will prevent certain diseases in a population, because we know what causes these diseases and we know that the chlorine treatment will remove these causes. We can predict that adding nicotinic acid to flour will practically eradicate pellagra because we know that the latter is a vitamin-deficiency disease. We know that vaccinating everyone with attenuated smallpox virus will eradicate smallpox because of its protective action in the body.

But we do not know how to prevent schizophrenia because there is no way of predicting who will get it. We could take extraordinary measures and force everyone to take large quantities of nicotinamide each day. This might well produce a marked decrease in schizophrenia over a period of years. But, we confidently predict that however good the idea might be, it will never be accepted. Think of the uproar the proposal would create in your community. Civil rights groups would form by the score. Anti-nicotinic acid groups for democratic action would march on the capital. Rumors would circulate that nicotinic acid causes baldness, hangnail and jaundice. At present it seems premature to get involved in this type of campaign to prevent schizophrenia.

Many suggestions have been made for preventing schizophrenia.

1. One suggestion is to find schizoid children and give them psychotherapy. Since most "schizoid" (quiet) children do not become schizophrenic,this prescription is useless. And even if

they were destined for this disease, psychotherapy wouldn't help.

2. Treat all disturbed children in out-patient clinics. This is no better than the suggestion above for no one has ever shown that schizophrenia can be prevented by psychotherapy of any sort. Of course, the suggestion would be helpful in creating a demand for more clinics, creating more jobs and increasing the professional treating force. All we are saying is that this would serve no useful purpose in preventing schizophrenia.

3. Love all your children equally. Since there is no useful definition of love, this prescription is of no value. Even if it could be valuable, there is much evidence that whether or not we love our children makes little difference. It is, of course, desirable that parents love their children for moral, ethical and many other reasons, but not because it will prevent them from becoming schizophrenic, for it won't.

4. Sterilization of schizophrenic patients. Even if this were morally and ethically advisable, it would not decrease the incidence, for, as we have shown earlier, most patients who develop schizophrenia come from normal parents.

5. Changing family structure. Some professionals say that the oldest child has the most stress since the parents are inexperienced and the child has the most responsibility. Others claim that the youngest is dominated by the older children. Alternately some claim that the parents wanted a girl to follow the boy or vice versa. And let us not forget the middle child who is said to be having difficulties because the parents concentrate their love and attention on the older and younger ones. No one has yet come up with any practical suggestions for altering the sex or the order in which a child is born in the family, nor is there any evidence that family structure has a bearing on schizophrenia. So even if we could change it, why try?

6. Reduce poverty. This is a very important function of society. Poverty is degrading and stifling to human energies and talents. Raising living standards is a worthwhile project in itself. So why look for reasons for tackling this great social problem other than it needs to be done? We have been told that eliminating poverty would reduce the incidence of schizophrenia, but we have found no connection between poverty and this disease. It seems likely, not that poverty breeds schizophrenia, but that badly treated schizophrenia leads to poverty. In

curing schizophrenia, therefore we might accomplish two things: get sick people well, and reduce poverty.

7. Decrease stress. Since there is little evidence that stress can produce schizophrenia, it will make little difference if stress is decreased. Almost anything is called stress these days. If the patient's mother's death precedes the onset of the disease, this is stress. If the patient happened to be moving from one city to another at a crucial time in his health history, this is stress. If we look upon mortality and morbidity as true measures of stress, however, we find there is less stress in many Western cultures than in primitive or undeveloped societies. Yet the incidence of schizophrenia remains the same throughout the world. Finally even if it were a significant factor, it is impossible to reduce stress quickly enough to do any one patient any good. Perhaps in several centuries stress will be under control. But, none of us will live long enough to benefit.

Since schizophrenia cannot be prevented, what can be done? Perhaps the day will come when malvaria tests, and other diagnostic tests still to be developed, will be as routine as TB tests are today. When that day comes, schizophrenia will no longer be the scourge it is now, and we will have come as close to prevention as possible.

Meanwhile it is possible to prevent chronic schizophrenia by early diagnosis and effective treatments. Preventive psychiatry is therefore:

1. Early diagnosis.
2. Adequate treatment.
3. Proper follow-up supervision.
4. Research.

Unfortunately, this is all we can offer until it becomes possible to predict who will become schizophrenic long before this happens. It is enough, however, to restore many patients to normal and productive lives at home and at work. There is much that can and should be done now.

RECOMMENDED READING

A. To understand what it is like to suffer schizophrenia

ANGYAL, A.: (1936) "Phenomena resembling lilliputian hallucinations in schizophrenia." *Arch. Neurol. Psychiat.* 36: 34–41.

ANON: (1850b) "Confessions of a patient after recovering from an attack of lunacy." *J. Psychol. Med.* 3: 388–399.

ANON: (1955) "An autobiography of a schizophrenic experience." *J. Abnorm. Soc. Psychol.* 51: 677–689.

BEERS, C. W.: (1908) *A Mind that Found Itself.* New York: Longmans, Green.

BOCKNER, S.: (1949) "The depersonalization syndrome: Report of a case." *J. Ment. Sci.* 95: 968–971.

BOISEN, A. T.: (1936) *The Exploration of the Inner World.* Chicago: Lillett, Clark.

BROWN, H. C.: (1937) *A Mind Mislaid.* New York: Dutton.

CONOLLY, J.: (1964) *The Indications of Insanity.* Dawsons of Pall Mall, London.

CUSTANCE, J.: (1952) *Wisdom, Madness and Folly.* New York: Pellegrini & Cudahy.

DAHL, R.: (1959) *Breakdown.* Indianapolis: Bobbs-Merrill.

DAVIDSON, D.: (1912) *Remembrance of a Religio-Maniac.* Stratford-on-Avon, England: Shakespeare Press.

FOY, J. G. :(1970) *Gone is Shadows' Child.* Logos International, Plainfield, New York.

FRASER, R. and W. SARGEANT: (1940–1941) "The subjective experiences of a schizophrenic illness: Personal records written at the end of the illness by some patients who were treated with insulin." *Character & Pers.* 9: 139–151.

HACKET, P.: (1952) *The Cardboard Giants.* New York: Putnam.

HENNELL, T.: (1938) *The Witnesses.* London: Davies.

JAMES, W.: (1902) *The Varieties of Religious Experience.* New York: Longmans, Green.

KRAUCH, E.: (1937) *A Mind Restored: The Story of Jim Curran.* New York: Putnam.

LEONARD, W. E.: (1939) *The Locomotive-God.* New York: Appleton-Century.

LORENZ, S. E. (1963) *And Always Tomorrow.* New York: Holt, Rinehart and Winston.

MACALPINE, I., and HUNTER, R. A.: (1956) *Schizophrenia, 1677: A Psychiatric Study of an Illustrated Autobiographical Record of Demoniacal Possession.* London: Dawson.

MERIVALE, H.: (1879) *My Experiences in a Lunatic Asylum.* London: Chatto & Windus.

MOORE, W. L.: (1955) *The Mind in Chains.* New York: Exposition Press.

NIJINSKY, R. (Ed.): (1936) *The Diary of Vaslav Nijinsky.* New York: Simon & Schuster.

O'BRIENT, B.: (1958) *Operators and Things: The Inner Life of a Schizophrenic.* Cambridge, Mass.: Arlington.

RAYMOND, E. (Ed.): (1946) *The Autobiography of David* —. London: Gollancz.

SCHREBER, D. P.: (1955) *Memoirs of My Nervous Illness.* (Ed. and trans. by I. Macalpine and R. A. Hunter.) London: Dawson.

SECHEHAYE, M.: (1951) *Autobiography of a Schizophrenic Girl.* New York: Grune and Stratton.

STEFAN, G.: (1967) *In Search of Sanity.* University Books, Inc., New Hyde Park, New York.

STUART, G.: (1953) *Private World of Pain.* London: Allen & Unwin.

SWEDENBORG, E.: (1839) *Concerning the Earths in Our Solar System which are called Planets.* Boston: Clapp.

SYMONS, A.: (1930) *Confessions: A Study in Pathology.* New York: Fountain Press.

VINCENT, J.: (1948) *Inside the Asylum.* London: Allen & Unwin.

WARD, M. J.: (1946) *The Snake Pit.* New York: Random House.

WECHSLER, J. A.: (1972) *In a Darkness.* New York: W. W. Norton and Co.

WELLON, A.:)1967) *Five Years in Mental Hospitals.* Exposition Press, New York.

B. *Theory and Treatment*

GOTTESMAN, I. I. and SHIELDS, J.: (1972) *Schizophrenia and Genetics.* Academic Press, New York.
HEACOCK, R. A. and POWELL, W. S.: (1972) "Adrenochrome and Related Compounds." *Progress in Medicinal Chemistry* 9, 275–240 Buttersworths, London.
KETY, S. S.; ROSENTHAL, D.; WENDER, P. H. and SCHULSINGER, F.: (1968) *The Transmission of Schizophrenia.* Oxford, England: Pergamon Press. Oxford, England.
PAULING, LINUS: (1968) "Orthomolecular Psychiatry." *Science* 160, 265–271.

C. *List of Publications, Canadian Schizophrenia Foundation, Regina, Saskatchewan*

1. Research and Troubled Children.
2. What to Do If You Have a Troubled Child.
3. How to Judge a Mental Hospital.
4. Which Treatment Should a Schizophrenic Seek?
5. Doctors Speak on the Orthomolecular Approach.
6. This is Schizophrenics Anonymous.
7. *Journal of Orthomolecular Psychiatry.* By subscription or by Membership in the Huxley Institute for Biosocial Research and the Canadian Schizophrenia Foundation.

INDEX